OSCEsmart

50 Medical Student OSCEs
in Paediatrics

Dr. Kunal Babla

Executive Consulting Editor:
Dr. Sam Thenabadu

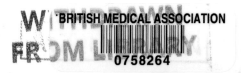

Ordering Information: Quantity sales. Special discounts are available on quantity purchases by corporations, associations, and others. For details, contact the publisher at the address above.

Orders by UK trade bookstores and wholesalers please visit www.scowenpublishing.com

Although every effort has been made to check this text, it is possible that errors have been made, readers are urged to check with the most up to date guidelines and safety regulations.

The authors and the publishers do not accept responsibility or legal liability for any errors in the text, or for the misuse of the material in this book.

Publisher's Cataloging-in-Publication data : OSCEsmart 50 medical student OSCEs in Paediatrics

ISBN-10: 0-9985267-3-8
ISBN-13: 978-0-9985267-3-7

CONTENTS

Message from the authors

Doctors of all seniorities can remember the stress of the OSCE but even more so the stress of trying to study and practice for the OSCEs. A multitude of generic undergraduate and postgraduate resources can be found on line but quality, quantity, and completeness of content can vary. The aim of the OSCESmart editorial team is to bring together specialty focused books that have identified 50 core stations encompassing the essential categories of history taking, examinations, emergency moulages, clinical skills and data interpretation with a strong theme of communications running through all the stations.

The combined experience of consultants, registrars and junior doctors to write, edit and quality check these stations, promises to deliver content that is appropriate to reach a standard we would expect of new junior doctors entering their foundation internship years and into core training. It is important to know that these stations are all newly written and based at the level of clinical competencies we would expect from these grades of doctors. Learning objectives exist for undergraduate curricula and for the foundation years, and the scenarios are based and written around these. What they are not, are scenarios that have been 'borrowed' from any medical school.

Preparation is the key to success in most things, but never more so than for the OSCEs and a candidate that hasn't practised will soon be found out. These books will allow you to practice relevant scenarios with verified checklists to learn both content and the generic approach. The format will allow you to practice in groups with one person being the candidate, one the actor and one the examiner. Each scenario finishes with three learning points. Picture these as are three core learning tips that we would want you to take away if you had only a couple of days left to the exam. These OSCE scenarios promise to be a robust revision aide for the student looking to recap and consolidate for their exams, but equally importantly prepare them for life in clinical practice.

I am immensely proud of this OSCESmart series. I have had the pleasure of working with some of the brightest and most dynamic young clinicians and educators I know, and I am sure you will find this series covering the essential clinical specialties a truly robust and invaluable companion in those stressful times of revision. I must take this opportunity to thank my colleagues for all their hard work but most of all to thank my wonderful wife Molly for her unerring love and support and my sons Reuben and Rafael for all the joy they bring me.

Despite the challenging times the health service finds itself in, being a doctor remains a huge privilege. We hope that this OSCESmart series goes some way to help you achieve the excellence you and your patients deserve.

Best of luck, Dr Sam Thenabadu

Introduction to OSCE Smart in Paediatrics

The beauty of Paediatrics lies in its variety. However, this variety can be daunting to medical students and junior doctors alike.

This book aims to help students and junior doctors prepare themselves for medical school OSCEs, as well as postgraduate exams such as MRCPCH or DCH clinical exams. Cases and scenarios have been carefully selected and written to challenge candidates and prepare you thoroughly for cases that commonly appear in exams at all levels.

The stations have been designed for you to practice in pairs or small groups, but also have central learning points that allow for reflection later, to allow you to maximise your performance in the real exam, or simply refresh your memory while working on the ward.

The book is split broadly into history taking, explanation, clinical examination and clinical skills. The stations cover a range of systems and scenarios designed to test and improve your communication, examination and key clinical skills.

History stations cover common complaints such as bronchiolitis and seizures, while the communications scenarios will challenge you to discuss breaking difficult news about critically ill children to their parents, or negotiate treatment plans. The full range of clinical examinations are covered and thoroughly examined with priceless tips on how to get the most out of your examination of young or uncooperative children. The practical stations will help you hone key clinical skills such as prescribing in paediatrics and administration of injectable medications.

This fantastic learning resource could not have been completed without the effort and dedication of all the contributing authors who have worked hard to ensure each station allows you to get the most out of your exam preparation. Our Consulting Editor, Sam Thenabadu has, as ever, been a source of wisdom and guidance throughout the process of completing this project and has our deepest gratitude. Perhaps most of all, thanks should go to all our colleagues and families who provided the support and encouragement we all needed to dedicate time and effort to producing this book.

Enjoy the book, enjoy your revision and good luck for your exams!

Kunal Babla

About the Authors

Dr Kunal Babla

Bsc(Hons) MBBS Msc MRCPCH MAcadMEd

ST6 Neonatal Medicine, London

Kunal graduated from the MBBS course at Guy's King's and St Thomas' School of Medicine in 2009, as well as gaining a BSc(Hons) in Anatomy. He went on to specialty training in Paediatrics in London, before taking up a Subspecialty Grid training post in Neonatal Medicine in 2016, where has developed a clinical and research interest in Neonatal Cardiology and haemodynamics.

As an accredited member of the Academy of Medical Educators, Kunal has a strong background in Medical Education, and has presented work at regional and national level. He has regular commitments as a Simulation Instructor and Newborn Life Support Instructor.

.

Dr Sam Thenabadu

MBBS MRCP DRCOG DCH MA Clin Ed FRCEM Msc (Paed) FHEA

Consultant Adult & Paediatric Emergency Medicine
Honorary Senior Lecturer & Associate Director of Medical Education

Sam Thenabadu graduated from King's College Medical School in 2001 and dual trained in Adult and Paediatric Emergency Medicine in London before being appointed a consultant in 2011 at the Princess Royal University Hospital. He has Masters degrees in Clinical Medical Education and Advanced Paediatrics.

He is undergraduate director of medical education at the King's College NHS Trust and the academic block lead for Emergency

Medicine and Critical Care at King's College School of Medicine. At postgraduate level he has been the Pan London Health Education England lead for CT3 paediatric emergency medicine trainees since 2011. Academically he has previously written two textbooks and has published in peer review journals and given numerous oral and poster presentations at national conferences in emergency medicine, paediatrics, medical education and patient quality and safety.

He has an unashamed passion for medical education and strives to achieve excellence for himself, his colleagues and his patients, hoping to always deliver this through an enjoyable learning environment. Service delivery and educational need not be two separate entities, and he hopes that those who have had great teachers will take it upon themselves to do the same for others in the future.

Co-authors

Dr Morium Akthar BSc (Hons) MBBS Msc (Paed) MRCPCH
ST8 Paediatrics, London

Dr Eleanor Bond BSc (Hons) MBBS MRCPCH
ST8 Paediatrics, London

Dr Sarah Davies BM (Hons) MA (Oxon) Experimental Psychology,
MRCPCH
ST4 Paediatrics, London

Dr Charlotte Doyle BSc (Hons) MBBS
ST1 Paediatrics, London

Dr Dionysios N. Grigoratos BSc(Hons) MBBS(Lon) MRCPCH
Paediatric Registrar, London

Dr Emily Haseler BM BCh MRCPCH
ST3 Paediatrics, London

Dr Sarah Hewett BSc(Hons) MBBS
ST2 Paediatrics, London

Dr Kathryn Smith MBChB Msc MRCPCH
ST5 Paediatrics, London

Dr Kirsten Thompson MBChB BMedSci
ST1 Paediatrics, London

Dr Lyndon Wells BMedSc (Hons) MBChB
ST2 Paediatrics, London

Abbreviations
ASD – Atrial Septal Defect
BNF – British National Formulary
BNFC – British National Formulary for Children
CAMHS – Child and Adolescent Mental Health Service
CRP – C-Reactive Protein
CT – Computed Tomography
CXR – Chest X-ray
DKA – Diabetic Ketoacidosis
ED – Emergency Department
EEG - Electroencephalogram
ESR – Erythrocyte Sedimentation Rate
FBC – Full Blood Count
FY1 Doctor – Foundation Year 1 Doctor
GBS – Group B Streptococcus
GP – General Practitioner
HIE – Hypoxic Ischaemic Encephalopathy
HIV – Human Immunodeficiency Virus
HR – Heart rate
IV - Intravenous
LDH – Lactate Dehydrogenase
LFT – Liver Function Test
LRTI – Lower Respiratory Tract Infection
MDI – Metered Dose Inhaler
MDT – Multidisciplinary Team
MRI – Magnetic Resonance Imaging
NAI – Non Accidental Injury
NBM – Nil by mouth
NICE – National Institute for Health and Care Excellence
PDA – Patent Ductus Arteriosus
PFO – Patent Foramen Ovale
PICU – Paediatric Intensive Care
PPROM – Preterm Prolonged Rupture of Membranes
PROM – Prolonged Rupture of Membranes
RR – Respiratory Rate
TSH – Thyroid Stimulating Hormone
U&E – Urea & Electrolytes
USS – Ultrasound Scan
UTI – Urinary Tract Infection
VSD – Ventricular Septal Defect

1. HISTORY - WITNESSED FIT

Candidate's Instructions:

A 10 year old boy called Paul has come into ED via ambulance with his father after witnessing him having a fit. Paul is currently sitting on a trolley with a GCS of 15.

You are the FY1 doctor in the paediatric team and have been asked to take a history.

With 2 minutes remaining the examiner will stop you, ask you to summarise back your findings and will ask you some direct questions.

Examiner's Instructions:

A 10 year old boy called Paul has come into ED via ambulance with his father after witnessing him having a fit. Paul is currently sitting on a trolley with a GCS of 15.

The FY1 doctor in the paediatric team has been asked to take the initial history.

After 6 minutes stop the candidate whatever stage they are at and ask them to summarise their findings and management plan.

Actor's Instructions:

You are the father of a 10 year boy, Paul, who you have brought to the Emergency Department after ringing an ambulance. You were making breakfast in the kitchen when you heard a thudding noise coming from upstairs. You ran upstairs to find Paul on the floor not responding to you and jerking all of his limbs. You also noted Paul has wet himself whilst you were ringing for an ambulance.

This kind of thing has never happened before and you didn't know what to do. The fit did not stop until the ambulance arrived and gave him some medication to make it stop. You think the whole episode lasted about 20 minutes. You don't know what they gave him but are worried he seems very sleepy and lethargic but is now responding to you.

You really want to know what tests need to be done and what can be done now. You are worried he could have epilepsy like his uncle. Paul usually lives with his mum but stays with you often. His mum dropped him off last night and was complaining he has been very clumsy recently especially in the morning when he is eating his cereal, but has not been unwell.

His immunisations are up to date and there are no developmental concerns. He has no known drug allergies and does not take any regular medication. He has not required any hospital admissions in the past. He was born at term by a normal delivery with no postnatal complications. He does not have any siblings and despite your separation you still get on well with his mother.

HISTORY- WITNESSED FIT

Task:	Achieved	Not Achieved
Introduces self		
Clarifies who they are speaking to and their relationship to child		
Elicits history from parent in a concise manner		
Elicits clear description of seizure		
Asks specifically about duration of seizure		
Asks about incontinence and tongue biting		
Establishes history of requiring medication to stop seizure		
Elicits history of being clumsy in the morning		
Asks about birth history		
Asks about past medical history		
Asks about drug history		
Establishes whether immunisations are up to date		
Asks about birth history		
Asks about developmental history		
Enquires about family history		
Elicits family history of epilepsy		
Asks about social history		
Responds appropriately to parental concerns about epilepsy		
Suggests appropriate investigations		
Summarises consultation & actions clearly		
Examiner's Global Mark	/5	
Actor / Helper's Global Mark	/5	
Total Station Mark	/30	

Learning Points

Take a clear chronological history when taking a collateral history regarding a possible witnessed seizure. Take a detailed account from the witness on what happened before, during and after the seizure. This will help clarify the type of seizure, and may inform your differential diagnoses for a non-traumatic loss of consciousness.

The importance of clear communication to reassure concerned parents especially after an episode of Status Epilepticus cannot be overstated. This also involves giving clear safety advice about minimizing risk of injury to the child in case of another seizure. Reassure parents that it is appropriate and important to call for an ambulance.

It is important to know how to investigate new or recurrent seizures. In this instance, basic blood tests and an ECG can be useful in ED to exclude non-neurological causes of loss of consciousness. Outpatient investigations such as EEG and MRI can be useful in determining the type or source of seizures. This can provide invaluable information with regards to treatment and prognosis.

2. HISTORY – SHORTNESS OF BREATH

Candidate's Instructions:

An 8 month old boy has been brought in by his parents with a 3 day history of cough reduced feeding and some difficulty in breathing.

You are the FY1 doctor in the paediatric team and have been asked to take a history and then summarise your findings back to the team.

With 2 minutes remaining the examiner will stop you, ask you to summarise back your findings and will ask you some direct questions.

Examiner's Instructions:

An 8 month old boy has been brought in by his parents with a 3 day history of cough reduced feeding and some difficulty in breathing.

The FY1 doctor in the paediatric team has been asked to take the initial history and then summarise their findings back to the team.

After 6 minutes stop the candidate whatever stage they are at and ask them summarise their findings and management plan.

Actor's Instructions:

Your 8 month old son, Sam, has been unwell for the last three days with a cough and runny nose. You live with your husband and three other children aged 3, 5 and 8, they are all usually fit and well. Your 3 year old has recently started nursery. He has had a cough and runny nose but has not had any difficulty in breathing like Sam.

Sam is much worse today as he is audibly wheezy. You noticed some slight in drawing of his ribs. He feels warm and has been very unsettled overnight. He usually sleeps very well. You are even more concerned as in triage the nurse commented that his oxygen levels were low at 94%. Sam has gone off his food but is drinking well and has not any diarrhoea or vomiting. He has no drug allergies, takes no regular medications, is passing urine and opening bowels normally with a normal number of wet and dirty nappies.

Your eldest son has asthma and you feel Sam needs inhalers to help him breathe. You feel he definitely needs to be admitted to be managed properly as he seems to be getting worse. It is only 3 weeks before Christmas and you want him to be well for his first Christmas. You feel antibiotics are the only thing that will make him better.

Sam was born at term by normal delivery. He had some breathing difficulties when he was first born. you remember he was breathing fast and needed antibiotics for 2 days but can't remember exactly why. His immunisations are up to date and there have never been any developmental concerns.

HISTORY – SHORTNESS OF BREATH

Task:	Achieved	Not Achieved
Introduces self		
Clarifies who they are speaking to and relationship to child		
Elicits history from parent in a concise manner		
Elicits onset and duration of illness		
Elicits history of cough and coryza		
Asks about shortness of breath		
Elicits history of wheeze / noisy breathing		
Asks about feeding and fluid intake		
Asks about history of fever		
Asks about contact with other unwell children		
Asks about past medical history		
Asks about drug history		
Establishes whether immunisations are up to date		
Asks about birth history		
Asks about developmental history		
Enquires about family history		
Asks about social history		
Suggests diagnosis of bronchiolitis		
Suggests appropriate investigations		
Summarises history and management plan concisely		
Examiner's Global Mark	/5	
Actor / Helper's Global Mark	/5	
Total Station Mark	/30	

Learning Points

Bronchiolitis is a viral infection caused most commonly by Respiratory Syncytial Virus. It occurs most during the September to March period in the UK, affecting mostly children under 12-18 months. As it is viral in nature, it resolves without specific medical intervention in the vast majority of cases. Some children will need supportive treatment in the form of oxygen, fluid or feeding support, and in the most severe cases, ventilatory support in a high-dependency or intensive care unit.

Remember to ask about specific signs and symptoms when taking a paediatric respiratory history. When considering Bronchiolitis these should include coryzal symptoms, cough, increased work of breathing, poor feeding, reduced wet nappies and fever.

Know the clinical indicators of increased work of breathing in young children. These include tachypnoea, head-bobbing, nasal flaring, subcostal/intercostal recession and grunting. In severe cases children may have apnoeic episodes. Always remember to check oxygen saturations in case there is an oxygen requirement.

3. HISTORY - FEBRILE ILLNESS

Candidate's Instructions:

A 3 month old boy has been brought in by his parents with a fever, reduced feeding and inconsolable crying.

You are the FY1 doctor in the paediatric team and have been asked to take a history and summarise your findings back to the team.

With 2 minutes remaining the examiner will stop you, ask you to summarise back your findings and will ask you some direct questions.

Examiner's Instructions:

A 3 month old boy has been brought in by his parents with a fever, reduced feeding and inconsolable crying.

The FY1 doctor in the paediatric team has been asked to take a history and then summarise their findings back to you.

After 6 minutes stop the candidate whatever stage they are at and ask them summarise their findings and management plan.

Actor's Instructions:

You and your husband have brought your 3 month old son, Roger, into the Emergency Department after an unsettled night. Roger was crying all night and neither of you were able to settle him. He has only been drinking about half of his usual amount. He keeps stopping while he is feeding as though he is in pain.

This morning you noted he was feeling very hot and his temperature measured 38.5°C in triage. You have not given him any Paracetamol or Ibuprofen, but kept him undressed without a nappy most of the morning as he seemed hot and uncomfortable. Whilst he was lying on the floor you noted he seemed more unsettled and in pain whilst passing urine. You have not noticed any rash, cough or coryzal symptoms. No one else is ill at home and you have not had any recent foreign travel.

He was born at 36 weeks and was treated with antibiotics due to prolonged rupture of membranes, but did not require any admission to SCBU or neonatal intensive care. His immunisations are up to date and he is due his second set in 2 days. You are worried that he might miss them.

He does not take any regular medication or have any known allergies. You are worried because he has been feeding and growing so well and he has never been off his bottles like this before. You are very concerned as your nephew had similar symptoms at this age and was in hospital for a week with meningitis.

HISTORY - FEBRILE ILLNESS

Task:	Achieved	Not Achieved
Introduces self		
Clarifies who they are speaking to and relationship to child		
Elicits history from parent in a concise manner		
Elicits history of febrile illness		
Elicits history of poor urine output		
Asks about feeding and fluid intake		
Asks about presence of rash		
Asks about symptoms associated with fever		
Asks about contact with other unwell people		
Asks about birth history		
Asks about past medical history		
Asks about drug history		
Establishes whether immunisations are up to date		
Asks about developmental history		
Enquires about family history		
Asks about social history		
Responds appropriately to parental concerns about epilepsy		
Suggests appropriate differentials including UTI		
Suggests appropriate investigations		
Summaries history and management plan concisely		
Examiner's Global Mark	/5	
Actor / Helper's Global Mark	/5	
Total Station Mark	/30	

Learning Points

It is important know how to assess a febrile illness in young children. The NICE guideline on assessment of a child with a febrile illness divides symptoms into:

Colour of skin, lips and tongue
Activity
Respiratory
Circulation and Hydration
Other: including rash and neurological signs

You can read the NICE guideline in more detail at: http://pathways.nice.org.uk/pathways/feverish-illness-in-children (National Institute for Health and Care Excellence 2016)

It is Important to establish a clear feeding/drinking history in young children, due to the risk of dehydration. Ask clearly how much they usually drink and how much they have had over the last 12-24 hours. You should also ask how many wet nappies they have had compared to usual.

Take a clear history of symptoms from the parents of a young child with a fever including indicators of the source of infection. This includes the timeframe of illness, coryzal symptoms and any rashes. Remember there are a vast number of different rashes in children. Purpura are seen in septicaemia and Henoch Schonlein Purpura. Viral erythematous maculopapaular rashes are seen in Slapped Cheek Disease (B19 parvovirus) and Roselea Infantum (herpes virus type-6).

4. HISTORY - FEBRILE CONVULSION

Candidate's Instructions:

A 3 year old girl is brought in by her mother via ambulance after an episode of shaking all over. The toddler is alert and active but miserable with a fever in triage.

You are the FY1 doctor in the Emergency Department and have been asked to take a history and then summarise your findings your findings back to the team.

With 2 minutes remaining the examiner will stop you, ask you to summarise back your findings and will ask you some direct questions.

Examiner's Instructions:

A 3 year old girl is brought in by her mother after an episode of shaking all over. The toddler is alert and active but miserable with a fever in triage.

The FY1 doctor in the paediatric team has been asked to take the initial history and then summarise their findings back to the team.

After 6 minutes stop the candidate whatever stage they are at and ask them summarise their findings and management plan.

Actor's Instructions:

You are the mother of a 3 year old girl, Freya. You rang an ambulance after she had an episode of being unresponsive and shaking all her limbs on the sofa. The whole episode lasted about 3-4 minutes in total. She was thrashing around abnormally, moving all four of her limbs. Her whole body seemed to be shaking like she was having a seizure. After she stopped shaking she was unresponsive and seemed a bit limp. She was still not herself when the paramedics arrived.

She was not at nursery today as she has had a fever for the last 3 days. She is off her food but drinking well. You are annoyed as you saw the GP yesterday who told you it was a viral throat infection that would settle.

Over the course of the day despite use of both Paracetamol and Ibuprofen her temperature was not coming down. She last had Paracetamol 4 hours ago and Ibuprofen 2 hours ago. She still had a temperature of 39°C at home just before the seizure happened. She has been miserable all day and is still hot. She is not her usual happy self in the Emergency Department.

Freya has a 6 year old brother who had a similar episode when he was 4 years old. You were told it was a febrile convulsion. You think your mother told you that you had a similar episode when you were a toddler. You know what a febrile convulsion is, but you are concerned as the shaking seemed much worse than it was in your son.

Freya does not take any regular medications, but has had 2 bouts of tonsillitis in the last year requiring antibiotics. Freya was born at term via elective C-section for breech position, but had no postnatal complications. She is developing well for her age with a good vocabulary and is dry by day. Freya does not have any known allergies, but does suffer from mild eczema.

HISTORY - FEBRILE CONVULSION

Task:	Achieved	Not Achieved
Introduces self		
Clarifies who they are speaking to and relationship to child		
Elicits history from parent in a concise manner		
Elicits history of fever prior to episode		
Elicits clear description of seizure		
Asks specifically about duration		
Asks about incontinence and tongue biting		
Elicits 3 day history of tonsillitis		
Asks about fluid intake		
Asks about birth history		
Asks about past medical history		
Asks about drug history		
Establishes whether immunisations are up to date		
Asks about developmental history		
Enquires about family history		
Establishes past family history of febrile convulsion in mother and brother		
Asks about social history		
Responds appropriately to parental concerns about seizure		
Suggests likely diagnosis of febrile convulsion		
Summaries history and management plan concisely		
Examiner's Global Mark	/5	
Actor / Helper's Global Mark	/5	
Total Station Mark	/30	

Learning Points

A febrile convulsion is characterised as a seizure in the presence of a fever and is most common between the ages of 6 months and six years. Viral illnesses associated with febrile convulsions include tonsillitis, otitis media and gastroenteritis, but it is important to exclude serious bacterial infections such as urinary tract infections and meningitis. A thorough, clear history will help you identify the underlying cause.

Take a clear chronological history when taking a collateral history regarding a possible witnessed febrile convulsion. Take a detailed account from the witness on what happened before, during and after the seizure, as well as how long it lasted or whether any specific treatment was needed.

Febrile convulsions are twice as common in males than in females and occur between 2%-4% of children. Be aware that risk factors for repeat seizures include, younger age at first seizure, earlier in infection at first seizure, family history of febrile convulsions or any past medical history of focal neurology or developmental delay.

5. HISTORY – HIGH BLOOD GLUCOSE

Candidate's Instructions:

The parents of an 8 year old boy presents to the Emergency Department with diarrhoea and vomiting. The triage nurse reports that he has sweet smelling breath and a high blood sugar reading of 30mmol/L.

You are the FY1 doctor in the paediatric team and have been asked to take a history and summarise your findings back to the team.

With 2 minutes remaining the examiner will stop you, ask you to summarise back your findings and will ask you some direct questions.

Examiner's Instructions:

The parents of an 8 year old boy presents to the Emergency Department with diarrhoea and vomiting. The triage nurse notes him to have sweet smelling breath and a high blood sugar reading of 30mmol/L.

The FY1 doctor in the Emergency Department has been asked to take a history and then summarise their findings back their senior.

After 6 minutes stop the candidate whatever stage they are at and ask them summarise their findings and management plan.

Actor's Instructions:

You have brought your son, Jordan, to the Emergency Department as he has become very lethargic due to ongoing diarrhoea and vomiting for the last 24 hours. The triage nurse commented on his sweet smelling breath, which you had not noticed yourself. You are worried about the high blood sugar reading she found in triage.

You are aware that over the last few weeks Jordan has been getting up at night to go the toilet and has been drinking a lot more than usual. You think he is looking thinner than he used to be as well. You wanted to see your GP to discuss his weight loss and getting up at night to go to the toilet, but haven't managed to organise an appointment yet.

Jordan is usually fit and well, his immunisations are up to date with no developmental concerns. He does not take any regular medications, does not have allergies that you know of and has had no previous hospital admissions. Jordan was born by a normal vaginal delivery, at term with no postnatal complications.

You have another child aged 5, Benjamin, who is usually fit and well, but has also had vomiting and diarrhoea. Benjamin is almost back to his usual happy and playful self. You are concerned that Jordan has got the same bug as Benjamin, but does not seem to be getting better as quickly.

The main reason that you have come to the Emergency Department was that your mother was at the house, who had diabetes diagnosed a few years ago. She checked Jordan's blood sugar and found it was reading 28. You are concerned what this means as you thought it would be low as he is unwell and not really eating much at the moment. The only people you know with high blood sugars are older people with diabetes like your mother.

HISTORY – HIGH BLOOD GLUCOSE

Task:	Achieved	Not Achieved
Introduces self		
Clarifies who they are speaking to and relationship to child		
Elicits history from mother in a concise manner		
Elicits history of polydipsia and polyuria		
Elicits history of new onset nocturia		
Elicits history of weight loss		
Elicits history of high blood sugar readings		
Asks about past medical history		
Asks specifically about other autoimmune or endocrine disorders		
Asks about drug history		
Establishes whether immunisations are up to date		
Asks about birth history		
Asks about developmental history		
Enquires about family history		
Elicits history of grandmother's Type 2 Diabetes		
Asks about social history		
Responds appropriately to parental concerns about diabetes		
Suggests likely diagnosis of Diabetic Ketoacidosis		
Suggests appropriate investigations		
Summaries history and management plan concisely		
Examiner's Global Mark	/5	
Actor / Helper's Global Mark	/5	
Total Station Mark	/30	

Learning Points

Type 1 Diabetes presents in a number of ways, but remember to explore evidence of the common signs and symptoms in a history. It is a challenging diagnosis to make without a previous history of known diabetes. Symptoms can be vague so eliciting longer-standing symptoms within the history can be vital. These may include excessive thirst, polyuria, unintended weight loss, lethargy or malaise. Children commonly present for the first time with evidence of DKA, and some may present in a critically ill condition requiring close monitoring or intensive care.

Remember when considering new onset of diabetes to look for evidence of other associated autoimmune conditions such as joint pain, thyroid illness and vitiligo.

Other possible differentials that could present with similar symptoms should be considered within the history. It is important to enquire about foreign travel and potential for exposure to viral illness (ie HIV).

6. HISTORY - SLOW WEIGHT GAIN

Candidate's Instructions:

A mother has brought her 14 month old baby girl to the Paediatric Outpatient Department. She was referred by her GP, who was concerned that her growth has been poor.

You are the FY1 doctor in the paediatrics team and have been asked to take the history, and then to summarise your findings to the team.

With 2 minutes remaining the examiner will stop you, ask you to summarise back your findings and will ask you some direct questions.

Examiner's Instructions:

A mother has brought her 14 month old baby girl to the Paediatric Outpatient Department. She was referred by her GP, who was concerned that her growth has been poor.

The FY1 doctor in the paediatric team has been asked to take the history and to summarise their findings back to the team.

Please show the candidate the growth chart if they ask for it. If not, please use it to facilitate discussion after the history has been taken.

After 6 minutes ask the candidate to conclude the discussion and ask them to summarise the history, and to discuss their management plan.

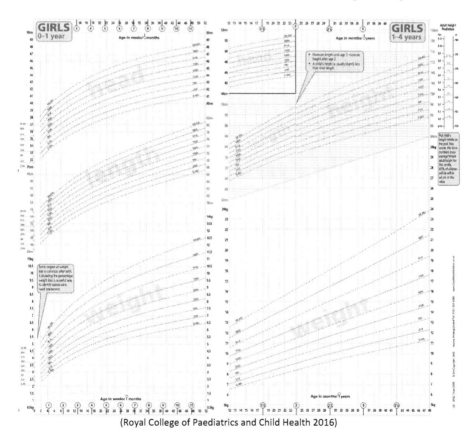

(Royal College of Paediatrics and Child Health 2016)

Actor's Instructions:

Your GP has referred your 14 month old daughter to the Paediatric Outpatient Clinic. The GP has been concerned that your daughter has not been growing very well. You first went to see your GP a few months ago because you were concerned that your daughter was smaller than your friend's child, who is two months younger.

Your daughter tends to get sick quite a lot. If anyone around her has a cold, she picks it up too. Her colds seem to go to her chest, and she has had a few courses of antibiotics for chest infections. She has been admitted to hospital three times with chest infections, needing antibiotics into the vein, and oxygen on one occasion. Even when she is well, she is a bit chesty. If specifically asks, she often has runny stool, which is quite foul smelling, and can be difficult to flush away.

She was exclusively breastfed until she was 6 months old, and then you started to introduce some solids. She is a fussy eater. She usually drinks a bottle of milk with breakfast, when she has some baby porridge. She has a snack in the morning with a bottle of milk, and then lunch – usually a little bit of meat, some vegetables and potato, although sometimes she doesn't want to finish her lunch. She has a bottle of milk in the afternoon, and usually has some of what you have for her dinner. She has another bottle of milk before bed.

She has had one admission to hospital with bronchiolitis. She needed oxygen for a couple of days. Otherwise, she has been well. She is up to date with her immunisations. There is no significant family history.

She is a quiet but content little girl. If asked, she sat without support at 11 months, but she cannot walk yet. She babbles and seems to know her name.

You live at home with your husband. She is your only child. Your husband's parents are around a lot and help you with childcare. Your husband smokes, but you do not. You are not known to social services.

HISTORY - SLOW WEIGHT GAIN

Task:	Achieved	Not Achieved
Introduces self		
Clarifies who they are speaking to and relationship to child		
Elicits history from mother in a concise manner		
Specifically asks about respiratory symptoms		
Specifically asks about GI symptoms, including diarrhoea and vomiting		
Specifically asks about infections		
Asks about feeding		
Asks about past medical history		
Asks about birth history		
Asks about family history		
Enquires about development		
Specifically asks whether the family is known to social services		
Identifies faltering growth from the growth chart		
Responds appropriately to parental concerns about growth		
Suggests appropriate differential diagnosis, including cystic fibrosis		
Suggests appropriate investigations, eg. baseline bloods, chest X-ray, urine dip, sputum culture, sweat test		
Summaries history and management plan concisely		
Management plan including MDT approach		
Suggests follow up to ensure weight gain improves		
Non-judgemental approach		
Examiner's Global Mark	/5	
Actor / Helper's Global Mark	/5	
Total Station Mark	/30	

Learning Points

Faltering growth (previously known as failure to thrive) is diagnosed when a child's weight crosses at least two centiles on the growth chart. It can helpful to think of causes of faltering growth as organic or non-organic, although there can be overlap. It is important to rule out organic causes, for example, coeliac disease, cow's milk protein intolerance, cystic fibrosis, hypothyroidism. You should also consider chronic or recurrent conditions, before considering non-organic causes, such as poor dietary intake, neglect, maternal mental health problems.

The multidisciplinary team is invaluable here. Consider the roles of the paediatrician, GP, health visitor, dietician, physiotherapist and others.

Remember to look for evidence of nutritional rickets, for example delayed dentition, frontal bossing, genu varum (bowed legs), developmental delay and cupping of epiphyses on X-ray.

7. HISTORY - HEADACHES

Candidate's Instructions:

A 14 year old girl has come to the Paediatric Outpatient Clinic with headaches, which she has been having for several months.

You are the FY1 doctor in the clinic, and have been asked to take a focussed history, and then to summarise your findings to the team.

With 2 minutes remaining the examiner will stop you, ask you to summarise back your findings and will ask you some direct questions.

Examiner's Instructions:

A 14 year old girl has come to the Paediatric Outpatient Clinic with headaches, which she has been having for several months. She has come with her mother, who allows her to give the history independently.

The FY1 doctor in the clinic has been asked to take the history, and then to summarise your findings to the team.

After 6 minutes ask the candidate to conclude the discussion and ask them to summarise the history, and to discuss their management plan.

Actor's Instructions:

You are 14 years old, and have been having headaches for about 6 months.

If specifically asked, the headaches start right in the middle of your forehead. They spread out towards your temples. They are not one sided. They feel like a dull ache. They happen once or twice a week, and are always the same. They come on gradually. There was no preceding head injury. Your vision seems ok – you have worn glasses for a couple of years, but there have been no recent changes. You have not noticed numbness, tingling or weakness anywhere. You have not had any vomiting. There is no aversion to bright lights, and your neck feels fine. They do not occur at a specific time of day. You have not noticed that they are worse when you cough, sneeze or stain. You haven't tried taking any painkillers. The severity is 6-7/10.

Otherwise, you are feeling ok. You have not had any fevers. You have not had any recent illnesses.

You do not have any other medical problems. You do not take any regular medications. You do not have any allergies. You don't think anyone else in the family has headaches. You don't know about your immunisations, or development as a baby. You started your period a year ago. They are regular. You are not sexually active.

You live at home with your mum and your three younger siblings. You have two brothers, aged 11 and 7, and a sister, aged 4. If asked, things are 'fine' at home. However, if encouraged, you reveal that you often have to help your mum with the work at home. You are worried because you think your mum is finding things really difficult. She hasn't said anything to you, but you think she is worried about money. She doesn't have anyone to help her. You're struggling with your school work. You feel tired, and the stress at home is making it difficult to concentrate.

HISTORY - HEADACHES

Task:	Achieved	Not Achieved
Introduces self		
Clarifies who they are speaking to and relationship to child		
Elicits history from child in a concise manner		
Asks about site of pain		
Asks about onset of the pain		
Asks about character of headaches		
Asks about radiation of the pain		
Asks about features of raised intracranial pressure, eg. worse on straining, worse in the morning, vomiting		
Asks about other associated symptoms, including fever, neck stiffness, photophobia		
Asks about the timing of the headaches		
Asks about exacerbating and relieving features		
Asks about severity of the pain		
Asks about past medical history		
Asks about family history		
Enquires about periods and sexual history		
Elicits concerning features from social history		
Responds appropriately to child's concerns		
Suggests appropriate differential diagnosis		
Suggests appropriate investigations		
Summarises history and management plan concisely		
Examiner's Global Mark	/5	
Actor / Helper's Global Mark	/5	
Total Station Mark	/30	

Learning Points

In any pain history, don't forget to ask about SOCRATES:
Site
Onset
Character
Radiation
Associated features
Timing
Exacerbating and relieving features
Severity

With headaches, it is vital to ask about red flags, so that you do not miss a brain tumour. It can be helpful to look at the Headsmart campaign for signs and symptoms of brain tumours in children of a variety of ages (HeadSmart 2016)

Be sensitive in your discussion of support available. Family structures have changed and many children and young adults may undertake the role of the carer. The child might be reluctant to accept help on behalf of her mother, and discussions between agencies should take place with the child and her mother.

8. HISTORY - UNEXPLAINED INJURY

Candidate's Instructions:

A mother brings her four month old baby to the local Emergency Department. He burned his arm.

You are the FY1 in the Emergency Department, and have been asked to see the child immediately as the nurse has concerns about the burn. You have been asked to take the history, and to summarise back to your team. You will need to discuss your next steps and management plan.

With 2 minutes remaining the examiner will stop you, ask you to summarise back your findings and will ask you some direct questions.

Examiner's Instructions:

A mother has brought her four month old baby to the local Emergency Department with a burnt arm.

The FY1 in the Emergency Department has been asked to see the child immediately as the nurse has concerns about the burn. They have been asked to take the history, and to summarise back to the team.

After 6 minutes ask the candidate to conclude the discussion and ask them to summarise the history, and to discuss their management plan. They will need to discuss their next steps, which should include how to escalate in this situation. Please prompt the candidate to suggest what they would do if the mother tries to leave.

Actor's Instructions:

You have brought your four month old baby to the Emergency Department because he burned his arm two days ago. He was sitting on his changing mat, and reached across and knocked over your cup of tea from the dining table while you were out of the room. He cried a lot at the beginning, but settled with a cuddle. It did not look like a bad burn, so you did not ask anyone to see him. The burn is over the back of his hand. You brought him today because it seems to be bothering him more, and you think it might be infected. You have just come for some antibiotics, and want to get back home.

Your baby was born at term. He is your only child, and it was an unplanned pregnancy. He was well after he was born, and you were discharged on the same day. He was difficult to feed initially, and sometimes he still takes a long time to feed, which can be difficult. Your scans were normal, and he has been well since he was born. He is on no regular medications, and has no allergies that you know of. You have not managed to get around to making an appointment for his immunisations, but you plan to at some point.

There is no family history of note. You have no medical problems.

In terms of development, he can smile, and can support his head. His hearing and vision seem fine, and he passed his newborn hearing check.

It's just the two of you at home. The baby's father left during the pregnancy, and you have not heard from him since. If asked, before he left he would hit you occasionally, but you never reported him. Everything at home is fine. You were seen by the 'young mums' midwife because you are 18, but you are not otherwise known to social services. Your parents live in Scotland, so are not around to help you, and you have been too busy to keep up with your friends since the baby was born. If probed, you are feeling isolated.

If the candidate summarises their history to you, you change your story, to say that the tea cup fell from a low table next to the changing mat.

You are unhappy to have to go through all of these details as you really just want antibiotics for your child. You become defensive if concerns are raised about the burn, and demand to leave once the antibiotics have been given. If challenged by security or the police you will concede and stay.

HISTORY - UNEXPLAINED INJURY

Task:	Achieved	Not Achieved
Introduces self		
Clarifies who they are speaking to and relationship to child		
Elicits history from parent in a concise manner		
Clarifies the history around the burn		
Asks about birth and past medical history		
Asks about immunisations		
Asks about developmental milestones		
Enquires about home situation		
Enquires specifically about other children at home		
Enquires about involvement with social services		
Summarises history to parent and checks details		
Explains concerns to parent in non-accusatory way and in clear simple terms		
Identifies concerning features in this history: delay in presenting, burn in unusual place, story not consistent with developmental age, change in story		
States 'duty of care to child' as overarching priority		
Explains need for the paediatric senior team to review patient today, and for admission for further investigation		
States will call security/police if tries to leave		
Summarises history and management plan concisely		
Does not collude with parent		
Remains calm		
Non judgmental approach		
Examiner's Global Mark	/5	
Actor / Helper's Global Mark	/5	
Total Station Mark	/30	

Learning Points

Be aware of certain patterns of injury which suggest non-accidental injury, for example burn to the back of the hand, immersion scalds, spiral fracture of the humerus, bruising in an identifiable pattern, e.g. bite mark, finger prints.

Known your milestones – non-accidental injury may present with an injury which could not be sustained at that stage in development. Always remember that under 3 months of age that babies simply can not roll, and any family that bring their child to the ED having 'rolled off the bed' needs to be challenged.

Remember to remain professional and honest. Secrecy can cause a situation to escalate later on. A detailed social history is particularly important in this station, and it is important that it is taken sensitively. Do not be judgemental, but do not collude with the parents. Your first duty of care is to the child and by explaining that both you and the parents have a shared objective progress can be made.

9. HISTORY - WEIGHT LOSS IN NEWBORN

Candidate's Instructions:

A 5 day old baby is referred into the Emergency Department by the community midwife, who is worried because the baby has lost 12% of his birth weight.

You are the FY1 doctor in the Paediatric team and have been asked to take the history, and then to summarise your findings to the team. You will need to explain your management plan to the mother.

With 2 minutes remaining the examiner will stop you, ask you to summarise back your findings and will ask you some direct questions.

Examiner's Instructions:

A 5 day old baby is referred into the Emergency Department by the community midwife, who is worried because the baby has lost 12% of his birth weight.

The FY1 doctor in the Paediatric team has been asked to take the history and to summarise their findings back to the team.

After 6 minutes ask the candidate to conclude the discussion and ask them to summarise the history, and to discuss their management plan.

Actor's Instructions:

You were seen at home by the community midwife for the 5 day postnatal check today. The midwife was concerned about your baby, because he has lost 12% of his birth weight. She told you to go to ED, and called ahead to say that you would be coming.

You have been exclusively breastfeeding your baby. He seems to be hungry a lot, and feeds all the time. It is difficult to settle him when he is off the breast. He feeds every hour, if not more often. He will fall asleep on the breast, but if moved, he wakes and starts to suck again.

He has passed urine twice in the last 24 hours, but has not opened his bowels. He has not been vomiting. You are concerned that he might be a bit more sleepy today. When he was awake yesterday, you thought that his eyes looked a bit yellow.

He was born at 39 weeks at this hospital following a normal delivery. He was fine after he was born, and went straight onto the breast. Your waters broke about 6 hours before he was born. You have been well in yourself, and have never heard of 'Group B Streptococcus'. You were discharged home the same day. He is your first baby. Your husband works during the day, but your mum is also around to help, and you feel well supported at home. You are not known to social services.

You have not given him formula, and you are very reluctant to do so. You have been told that formula can be harmful for babies. If questioned further, you become tearful, and say that you would feel like a failure as a mum if you were unable to provide enough milk for your baby. However, with clear and empathetic explanation, you would agree to give formula.

HISTORY - WEIGHT LOSS IN NEWBORN

Task:	Achieved	Not Achieved
Introduces self		
Clarifies who they are speaking to and relationship to child		
Elicits history from mother in a concise manner		
Asks about feeding		
Asks specifically about urine output		
Asks about any other maternal concerns		
Asks about pregnancy and antenatal screening		
Asks about birth history		
Asks about risk factors for sepsis		
Asks about past medical history of child		
Asks about social history		
Identifies features which suggest that breastfeeding has not been successfully established		
Identifies that 12% weight loss in a newborn in concerning and required admission		
Explains that the baby needs to be admitted for investigations and feeding support		
Explains the need for additional feed in this case in clear, simple terms		
Reassures mother that formula is not harmful for her baby		
Responds appropriately to mother's concerns about feeding		
Summarises history and management plan concisely		
Suggests appropriate investigations: U&Es, bilirubin		
Empathetic approach towards mother		
Examiner's Global Mark	/5	
Actor / Helper's Global Mark	/5	
Total Station Mark	/30	

Learning Points

Many babies will lose some weight in the first week, but more than 10% weight loss is concerning and requires admission for investigation and feeding support. Don't forget to ask about the birth history, asking specifically about the presence of Group B Streptococcus, prolonged rupture of membranes, maternal fever or infection and prematurity – all place infants at risk of perinatal infection.

Remember the effects of poor feeding include not just weight loss, but dehydration, poor urine output, hypernatraemia, jaundice and hypoglycaemia.

Clear, empathetic communication in this case can help you to negotiate a management plan for the baby which the mother is happy with. It is important that she does not feel as though she has been forced to do something that she did not want to do.

10. HISTORY – SPEECH DELAY

Candidate's Instructions:

A three year old is referred to the Paediatric Outpatient Department by the GP, who is concerned that the child has not started to talk yet.

You are the FY1 doctor in the clinic and have been asked to take the initial history, and to summarise your findings back to the team.

With 2 minutes remaining the examiner will stop you, ask you to summarise back your findings and will ask you some direct questions.

Examiner's Instructions:

A three year old is referred to the Paediatric Outpatient Department by the GP, who is concerned that the child has not started to talk yet.

The FY1 doctor in the paediatric team has been asked to take the history and to summarise their findings back to the team.

After 6 minutes ask the candidate to conclude the discussion and ask them to summarise the history, and to discuss their plan for investigations and management.

Actor's Instructions:

Your GP referred you into the clinic today with your son, who is three. You went to see the GP 6 weeks ago because you were worried that he is not yet speaking. You had wondered for a while whether his speech was a bit slow, but you really noticed it when you caught up with a friend and her two-and-a-half year old daughter recently. Your friend's daughter's speech seemed much clearer than your son's.

Your son was born at 37 weeks. He is generally a very healthy, happy boy. He has had a few coughs and colds, and a he had a tummy bug last year, but he has no long terms medical problems and takes no regular medication. He is up to date with his immunisations. He is an only child. There is no family history of speech problems.

In terms of development, he smiled at 6 weeks. He sat on his own at 8 months. He started to walk at 13 months, and ran by 18 months. He can now climb steps with one foot on each step. He loves to scribble, and if asked, can scribble circles. He can feed himself with a fork, and plays well with other children. You have no concerns about his vision.

With regards to his speech, he seems to understand what you say. He knows his name. He began to babble at around 7 or 8 months. He is a happy boy, and laughs a lot. He can use about 20 single words, but he does not seem able to put them together. He follows simple instructions, and can identify different animals from picture books if asked. He passed his newborn baby hearing screen, and you do not think that he has problems with his hearing.

You live at home with your son and your husband. Your husband is French, and you speak both English and French at home, because you want your son to be able to speak both languages. You and your husband both work, so your son spends time with the nanny during the day. You are not known to social services.

HISTORY – SPEECH DELAY

Task:	Achieved	Not Achieved
Introduces self		
Clarifies who they are speaking to and relationship to child		
Elicits history from mother in a concise manner		
Asks about gross motor development		
Asks about fine motor development		
Asks about social development		
Asks about expressive speech development		
Asks about receptive speech development		
Enquires about hearing		
Enquires about vision		
Asks about birth history		
Asks about past medical history		
Enquires about newborn hearing screen		
Asks about family history		
Asks about social history		
Responds appropriately to parent's concerns		
Identifies that this is an isolated speech delay		
Gives a differential diagnosis, including hearing loss, learning difficulties, autism, exposure to more than one language, emotional deprivation and neglect		
Summarises history and management plan concisely		
Management plan to include a hearing test and referral to SALT		
Examiner's Global Mark	/5	
Actor / Helper's Global Mark	/5	
Total Station Mark	/30	

Learning Points

With speech delay, always think about poor hearing, and consider referral for an audiology assessment. Routine hearing tests are done soon after birth, occasionally at the 2 year assessment and always at the age 4 preschool assessment but these children can be referred at any stage for testing.

With any type of developmental delay, remember to ask about all four domains of development; gross motor, fine motor, speech & hearing and social skills. Delay in two or more domains can be classed as "Global Developmental Delay".

Think about the support that this child and family might need going forwards – clearly the GP, community paediatrician and SALT teams will be invaluable. He might also need help with schooling. If there are concerns regarding emotional deprivation and neglect, then social services must be involved. Be aware that he may not need any intervention, as speech delay associated with exposure to more than one language is not in itself abnormal.

11. HISTORY – ACCIDENTAL POISONING

Candidate's instructions

Molly is a three year old girl who was brought to the Emergency Department by her father, as she has accidentally ingested an unknown amount of 'Calpol' paracetamol suspension.

You are the FY1 doctor in Paediatric ED. The team ask you to take a history from Molly's father and explain any management that might be required in the Emergency Department.

Molly has normal observations and is happily playing in the waiting room with her mother and brother, who have just arrived.

With 2 minutes remaining the examiner will stop you, ask you to summarise back your findings and will ask you some direct questions.

Examiner's Instructions

The candidate is a FY1 doctor in Paediatric ED. They have been asked to take a history and explain any management that might be required in the ED to the father of Molly, a three year old girl who has accidentally ingested an unknown amount of 'Calpol' paracetamol suspension. Molly's observations are normal, and she is happily playing.

The parent will express some anger if blood tests, cannulation or N-Acetylcysteine are suggested; however, if the candidate appropriately explains the potential harmful effects of accidental paracetamol overdose, the parent will calm down and express concern instead.

After 6 minutes ask the candidate to conclude the discussion and ask them to summarise the history, and to discuss their plan for investigations and management.

Actor's instructions

You found Molly in the kitchen two hours ago, with Calpol all over her herself, her clothes and the floor. You had left her colouring quietly downstairs for a couple of minutes to put her 10 month old brother down for a nap after giving him a dose of Calpol, as he's been grizzly with a temperature today.

Your wife and yourself normally keep all medicine on a high shelf of a cupboard, but in your rush to put her brother in his cot you must have left the open bottle on the kitchen countertop. When you came downstairs minutes later, it seems Molly had pushed a chair up alongside the kitchen surface and climbed up to retrieve it. You didn't even know she knew how to do this!

It's difficult to tell how much Calpol Molly might have ingested, as so much of it was over her face, hands, clothes and the floor, but it was a new bottle opened this morning and there's now almost nothing left in it. You called your GP for advice, who told you to attend ED immediately, which you have done.

Molly was born at term and has always been a healthy child; she is not unwell currently, and has been happy and playful since drinking the Calpol, with no vomiting. You live at home with your wife and 10 month old son. Your wife is a solicitor, and you work from home as a graphic designer. Both children go to nursery three days a week. Molly has no allergies or regular medication, there is no family history of note, and you have never been known to social services.

You aren't really sure why you need to be here, and if the candidate expresses a need to perform blood tests, cannulation, or possibly give IV medications you become angry - Molly is so well compared to the other children in the waiting area, and it's only Calpol which is pretty harmless. If they appropriately explain the potential harmful effects of Calpol ingestion, you quickly calm down and simply want to know what will be done to make it as painless as possible for Molly. If health visitor referral is mentioned, you have no problem with this.

HISTORY – ACCIDENTAL POISONING

	Achieved	Not Achieved
Introduces self		
Clarifies who they are speaking to and relationship to child		
Elicits timing of paracetamol ingestion		
Tries to quantify potential volume of suspension ingested (i.e. how much was in the bottle initially, how much was left)		
Elicits circumstances of paracetamol ingestion (i.e. child unattended, bottle left open by accident)		
Enquires about any immediate symptoms / vomiting		
Checks Molly has no intercurrent illness		
Asks about past medical history		
Asks about drug history		
Asks about immunisations		
Enquires about social history, including whether family are known to social services		
Explains concerns to parent in non-accusatory way and in clear, simple terms		
Explains potentially harmful effects of accidental paracetamol overdose above toxic dose of 75mg/kg		
Explains need for blood tests +/- cannula at 4 hours post-ingestion		
Responds appropriately to parent's concerns		
Discusses use of Ametop / EMLA / play therapy in making phlebotomy / cannulation as pain-free as possible		
Explains that dependent on blood test results, may need to start IV medication (N-acetylcysteine) in ED and be admitted		
Explains need for health visitor referral		
Discusses importance of a locked medicine cabinet now Molly is able to access kitchen countertop		
Summarises history and management plan concisely		
Examiner's global mark	/5	
Actor's global mark	/5	
Total Station Mark	/30	

Learning Points

Paracetamol suspension is widely used, and as it is sweetened it smells and tastes nice to young children – if they are able to get hold of an open bottle they will typically drink it, and so it is responsible for a relatively large proportional of accidental overdoses seen in Paediatric ED. Considering the number of intentional paracetamol overdoses also seen in Paediatric ED (typically in older children and teenagers), it is essential to both know and be able to explain the management of paracetamol overdose in the ED.

It can be very difficult to quantify exactly how much of any medication has been ingested by a child, for multiple reasons; parents are often unsure how much medication was in a bottle / packet to begin with, liquid suspensions tend to end up everywhere (over the child, the floor and the furniture), parents may not be able to tell you what strength tablets / suspension are, and the child is unlikely to give a reliable collateral history to tell you whether they actually swallowed anything, or spat it out. As a result we always work on the 'worst case scenario' of maximum possible ingestion, and determine management from there.

For this case, management should include:

Blood tests for paracetamol level, U&Es, LFTs and coagulation taken 4 hours after ingestion, with Ametop / EMLA and distraction or play therapy to make the process less distressing.

If the paracetamol level plots above the treatment line for N-acetylcysteine (NAC) on the British National Formulary for Children (BNFC) chart, start NAC in Paediatric ED and admit to the ward to continue treatment.

Advice to parents about storing medications safely with increasingly mobile and inquisitive children, as well as a health visitor referral, in view of an accidental overdose in a young child. Bear in mind that a three year old may be difficult to cannulate again after initial phlebotomy, should her paracetamol level come back high enough to require NAC, so it may be wise to put a cannula in whilst taking the initial blood tests.

12. HISTORY – DELIBERATE SELF HARM

Candidate's instructions

Alice is a twelve-year old girl who has been bought in to ED by her mother, after school noticed numerous cut marks on her forearms.

You are the FY1 doctor in Paediatric ED. The team have seen Alice with her mother and have dressed her forearm injuries, which are superficial and not of medical significance.

They ask you to speak to Alice without her mother present in order to assess her suicide risk. Both Alice and her mother have agreed to this.

With 2 minutes remaining the examiner will stop you, ask you to summarise back your findings and will ask you some direct questions.

Examiner's Instructions

The candidate is an FY1 doctor in Paediatric ED. They have been asked to assess the suicide risk of Alice, a 12 year old girl who has been brought to the ED by her mother after school noticed numerous cut marks on her forearms.

Alice has been seen with her mother already; her injuries are superficial, not of medical significance, and have been dressed. Both Alice and her mother have agreed that Alice should speak to a doctor on her own.

Alice is quiet and shy, but will open up and answer all questions asked if the candidate communicates empathetically.

After 6 minutes ask the candidate to conclude the discussion and ask them to summarise the history, and to discuss their plan for investigations and management.

Ask them:
1.   What do you think Alice's risk of suicide is, and why?
2.   What would be your next steps in management?

Actor's instructions

Your teacher noticed the cuts on your arms earlier and told your Mum about it. You told your Mum that you cut your arms deliberately, so she brought you to the ED to have your arms looked at.

You've always been very healthy and have never even been to a hospital before. You are shy and quiet, have never had a boyfriend, and have a really good group of friends. You enjoy school, but are finding Year 8 stressful as the work is harder; you are worried you might start to get lower grades, like B's and C's, and then your teachers and parents will be disappointed.

You live with your Mum, Dad, and 8 year old brother. Recently, Mum and Dad have been arguing a lot about things like the washing up and the laundry; they never hit each other or say swear words, but they didn't used to argue like this and you're worried that they might get divorced like some of your friend's parents. Your parents are always loving towards you and your brother, but you wish they wouldn't argue so much. You used to be really happy but now you often cry at home, and don't sleep as well as you used to. You haven't talked to your friends about it because they're upset about their own parents splitting up, and you're worried you might upset them more.

You used some scissors from your art box to cut your arms last night – you didn't plan to do it and have never done anything like this before, but you were upset after hearing your parents argue and somehow it made you feel better. You didn't mean to hurt yourself by doing it. You find your Mum easy to talk to, but didn't tell her or anyone else because you didn't think it was a big deal. You didn't expect anyone to notice the cuts or be so worried about them, and are quite embarrassed to be here.

You have never thought about killing yourself, and have never made any plans to do so. You don't have any plans to cut yourself again, but you are worried how you will cope with Mum and Dad arguing, as well as the stress of schoolwork. If the candidate asks if you think you would like someone (e.g. CAMHS, school counsellor) to talk to regularly, you really like this idea.

You will be quiet, answer questions briefly and make little eye contact initially. If the candidate speaks to you softly, and is empathetic, then you will engage with them much more, making eye contact and answering their questions fully.

HISTORY – DELIBERATE SELF HARM

	Achieved	Not Achieved
Introduces self		
Clarifies identity of patient		
Checks patient is still happy to talk without mother present		
Elicits what cuts were made with, when, and how		
Elicits intention of making cuts		
Asks about possible depressive symptoms (e.g. low mood, anhedonia, sleep, appetite)		
Asks about school; does she enjoy it? How is school performance? Does she find it stressful?		
Asks about friendship group / social support		
Ask about home life		
Clarifies that parents arguing does not pose any concern regarding abuse / domestic violence		
Asks specifically if she had suicidal intentions when self-harming		
Clarifies whether she has ever had suicidal ideation		
Uses age-appropriate language and terminology		
Responds empathetically to patient's emotional state		
Asks patient if there's anything that particularly worries her / that she thinks would help		
Summarises history back to patient		
Correctly assesses suicide risk as low		
Explains rationale for assigned suicide risk (e.g. intent, suicidal ideation, plans, protective factors)		
Demonstrates understanding of need to involve CAMHS and/or counselling services		
Demonstrates understanding of need to involve family (and possibly school) in future management		
Examiner's global mark	/5	
Actor's global mark	/5	
Total Station Mark	/30	

Learning Points

Speaking to the child without parents or guardians present can yield very important information. Feelings and emotions, home life, motives for self-harming actions, or other issues such as those surrounding boyfriends/girlfriends and/or sexual history can be very difficult for many children to discuss in front of the adults who care for them. In situations where it is important that the child fully discloses information about any of these areas, you should always attempt to speak to the child both with and without a parent or guardian present.

Stressors in childhood often arise from issues with home life, school, friendship group and relationships. To fully explore a self-harm history in a child you need ask specifically about these areas, as well as asking if there's anything else they are finding upsetting or stressful.

Child and Adolescent Mental Health Services (CAMHS) are integral in helping to support young children with self-harming behaviour and psychiatric conditions. However, when devising management plans it is important to involve all relevant parties – including school, and family – to ensure a holistic approach where the child is appropriately supported in all areas of their life.

13. HISTORY – LOSS OF CONSCIOUSNESS

Candidate's instructions

Jennifer is 13 year old girl who has been brought to ED by school, after she fainted in class; her mother has been informed she is in ED and is on her way.

You are the FY1 doctor in Paediatric ED. The team ask you to take a history from Jennifer, then discuss your findings.

Heart rate, respiratory rate, temperature and blood pressure are all normal. Jennifer looks well, and feels fine in herself.

With 2 minutes remaining the examiner will stop you, ask you to summarise back your findings and will ask you some direct questions.

Examiner's Instructions

The candidate is an FY1 doctor in Paediatric ED. They have been asked to take a history from Jennifer, a 13 year old girl who has been brought to ED by school after she fainted in class. Jennifer's observations are normal, and she looks and feels well.

Jennifer is happy and chatty, and will answer any question she can; she doesn't know much about her family history, or whether she had any health problems when she was younger.

After 6 minutes ask the candidate to conclude the discussion and ask them to summarise the history, and to discuss their plan for investigations and management.

Ask them:
1.   Please tell me what differential diagnoses you are considering.
2.   What advice would you give Jennifer and her parents?

Actor's instructions

You fainted in Biology class earlier today. The teacher was dissecting a frog whilst the class were stood up watching. You were ok for the first 10 minutes, but then you started to feel a bit light-headed, dizzy and sick. Your heart was racing and you remember your vision getting blurry around the edges; the next thing you remember, you were lying on the classroom floor with everyone looking at you!

Your classmates say you looked really pale just before you fainted, but a friend caught you as you fell and you didn't bump your head. They say you fainted for only a few seconds, and your limbs didn't twitch or anything like that. You remember everything from when you woke up, and you felt fine after you'd sat down for a few minutes and had some water, but because this has happened before your teacher brought you to ED.

The other time this happened was six months ago when you were stood up in Home Economics class watching the teacher, and the room was really hot because all the ovens were on. You felt exactly the same that time as well – dizzy, blurry vision, feeling sick - but you sat down until you felt better and didn't go to hospital.

You haven't been sick at all recently, and you feel absolutely fine now. You eat healthily and do bit of sport, but you don't watch what you eat and haven't lost any weight. You don't know anything about your past medical history. You live with your Mum and your 15 year old sister; your parents divorced when you were young and you see your Dad on weekends. You're happy with your family, school, and friends. You don't know anything about your family's medical history. You don't take any medicines or have any allergies.

You are happy, chatty and will answer any questions you can; but you don't know about family or personal medical history. You aren't worried about fainting, but it would be nice to be able to stop it happening.

HISTORY – LOSS OF CONSCIOUSNESS

	Achieved	Not Achieved
Introduces self		
Clarifies identity of patient		
Elicits clear history of pre-faint symptoms (feeling light-headed, dizzy, blurring vision)		
Elicits clear history of faint itself (duration, any abnormal movements, any injury sustained)		
Elicits clear history of post-faint (any amnesia, how long it took to return to normal)		
Asks about associated cardiac symptoms (palpitations, chest pain, colour change)		
Asks about associated neurological symptoms (aura, abnormal movement, post-ictal)		
Asks about intercurrent illness		
Asks about past medical history		
Clarifies history of previous fainting episode		
Asks about family and social history		
Asks about patient's ideas / concerns		
Uses age-appropriate language and terminology		
Summarises history back to patient		
Offers sensible differential diagnosis e.g. vasovagal syncope, prolonged QT, atypical seizure		
Recognises need for ECG		
Recognises need for lying & standing BP		
Recognises need for full cardiovascular and neurological examination		
Recognises need to attempt to obtain collateral history from a witness, e.g. from the teacher		
Recognises need for collateral history from mother regarding past medical history and family history (e.g. sudden death, cardiac and neurological history)		
Examiner's global mark	/5	
Actor's global mark	/5	
Total Station Mark	/30	

Learning Points

Causes of loss of consciousness in children are varied; whilst vasovagal syncope is the most common, as was the case here, other cardiac and neurological causes must always be considered. As such, all patients presenting with loss of consciousness must be asked about personal cardiac and neurological symptoms, as well as personal and family history of cardiac and neurological illness.

In particular, when taking a history remember to ask about any family history of sudden death. Whilst it can feel like a frightening question to ask parents, it significantly raises clinical suspicion of a genetic predisposition to prolonged QT syndrome. As this is a potentially preventable cause of sudden young adult death, which in high-risk cases can be managed with an implantable cardioverter defibrillator, it is a particularly important point to cover in history.

When examining and investigating these patients, they require at least cardiac and neurological exams, baseline observations including a blood glucose reading, an ECG, and lying and standing blood pressures. In any girl of childbearing age a pregnancy test should be performed. Other investigations such as EEG, echocardiogram and CT/MRI imaging of the brain may be required, dependent on history, but this level of investigation would be expected to be discussed with a senior or specialist first.

14. HISTORY – NEONATAL FLOPPY EPISODE

Candidate's instructions

Oscar is a three week old baby boy who has been brought to ED by his parents, after he had a floppy episode whilst feeding.

You are the FY1 doctor in Paediatric ED. The team ask you to take a history of the event from Oscar's mother. Oscar has normal observations, and the Paediatric nurse tells you he looks alert and active at triage.

With 2 minutes remaining the examiner will stop you, ask you to summarise back your findings and will ask you some direct questions.

Examiner's Instructions

The candidate is an FY1 doctor in Paediatric ED. They have been asked to take a history from the mother of Oscar, a three week old boy. His parents have brought him to the ED after he had a floppy episode whilst feeding. Oscar's observations are normal, and there are no acute clinical concerns.

The parent will express distress that Oscar could have died, and will want to know what can be done to make sure this doesn't happen again.

After 6 minutes ask the candidate to conclude the discussion and ask them to summarise the history, and to discuss their plan for investigations and management.

Ask them:
1.   Please tell me what differential diagnoses you are considering, and why.
2.   What would be your next steps in management?

Actor's instructions

You are Oscar's mother; he is you and your partner's first baby. You have rushed him to the ED because he had a floppy episode whilst feeding. You are shaken up, and on the verge of tears.

Your pregnancy was unremarkable, with normal scans and blood tests; this was a relief, after you and your partner suffered a miscarriage last year. He was born in hospital by normal vaginal delivery at 39 weeks. Your waters broke 6 hours before he was born, you had no temperature or IV antibiotics during labour, and you have never been told you have Group B Streptococcus. Oscar didn't require any resuscitation or neonatal unit care, and you were both discharged home the next day.

You have been breastfeeding Oscar since birth; his birth weight was 3.2kg, and he weighs 3.5kg now. He normally feeds on the breast every 2-3 hours, for 20 minutes. On this occasion Oscar had been feeding for around 15 minutes when you noticed he had stopped sucking – you looked down to see he was much floppier than normal. He seemed slightly pale, but you don't remember him looking blue; you picked him up, shouted for your partner, and blew in his face. He then vomited up a small amount of milk and gave a cry, before settling down as he normally would after a feed. The whole episode probably lasted 10-15 seconds, but felt much longer.

Oscar has been his normal self in the two hours since this happened, but you are now scared to feed him again – you want to know what you can do to stop this happening again, as at the time you and your partner both felt at the time that Oscar might die. Neither of you are happy to go home until you are certain this won't happen again. You and your partner are not related, and you are not married but live together; you both work as civil servants, and have no significant past medical history.

Other than today's floppy episode, Oscar has been a very healthy baby and has no current signs of illness. He has never had a floppy episode before, although vomits a small amount of milk after each feed which you were initially worried about; however, your health visitor reassured you that it was normal, particularly as he is gaining weight well.

HISTORY – NEONATAL FLOPPY EPISODE

	Achieved	Not Achieved
Introduces self		
Clarifies who they are speaking to and relationship to child		
Elicits a clear history of floppy episode		
Clarifies whether any colour change during episode		
Clarifies resolution of episode (how long, what action was taken / needed)		
Elicits pregnancy and birth history		
Elicits any risk factors for sepsis (e.g. GBS, PROM, pyrexia)		
Takes a feeding history (e.g. how long, how often)		
Elicits past medical history, including appropriate weight gain		
Asks about other signs / symptoms of intercurrent illness (e.g. pyrexia, lethargy, not waking for feeds, cough / cold)		
Elicits family history (including consanguinity)		
Elicits social history		
Uses appropriate lay terminology		
Asks about mother's ideas / concerns / expectations		
Responds empathetically to mother's emotion and concerns		
Summarises history back to mother		
Considers sensible differential diagnosis (e.g. normal baby, reflux, sepsis, cardiac, metabolic, trauma, seizure)		
Is able to appropriately justify differential diagnoses offered		
Recognises importance of physical examination +/- prolonged observation to aid diagnosis and reassure parents		
Recognises need to discuss management with a senior		
Examiner's global mark	/5	
Actor's global mark	/5	
Total Station Mark	/30	

Learning Points

Sometimes it can be very difficult to determine exactly what causes a floppy episode in a baby, or whether it's anything to worry about. In a baby who seems well, but where the cause or the history isn't certain, a pragmatic management plan often involves simply admitting the baby and parent for observation. This may not offer any more information regarding the underlying cause of the episode, but can help parents to feel much less anxious about taking their baby home.

In babies of this age, sepsis is a significant cause for concern; they are still at risk of late Group B Streptococcal (GBS) sepsis, and have not yet started their programme of childhood immunisations. Because of this, we always make sure to ask about risk factors for infection being acquired around the time of labour:
Did the mother have prolonged rupture of membranes (PROM) of more than 24 hours?
Was she a known carrier of GBS (a positive swab or urine result during pregnancy, or a previous baby with invasive GBS disease)?
Did she have a pyrexia of 39°C or more during labour?
Were the obstetric team otherwise worried enough about infection in mother to give her IV antibiotics during labour?

In addition to sepsis, other pathologies that result in babies presenting to ED in the first few weeks of life – either actively unwell, or just 'not quite right' – are cardiac causes, particularly duct-dependent congenital heart defects, metabolic causes, and trauma / Non-accidental injury (NAI). You must consider all of these when taking a history about a child of this age.

15. HISTORY – NON-TRAUMATIC BRUISING

Candidate's instructions

Ben is a two year old boy who has been brought to ED by his mother, as he has developed bruising on his arms and stomach overnight.

You are the FY1 doctor in Paediatric ED. The team ask you to take a history from Ben's mother as this is the third time she has bought him to the Emergency Department in two weeks.

The triage nurse confirms that Ben has multiple large bruises on his abdomen arms, and has normal observations; he looks tired but relatively well.

With 2 minutes remaining the examiner will stop you, ask you to summarise back your findings and will ask you some direct questions.

Examiner's Instructions

The candidate is a junior doctor in Paediatric ED. They have been asked to take a history from the mother of Ben, a two year old boy. His mother has brought him to the ED with bruising on his arms and stomach that has developed overnight. Ben's observations are normal, and there are no acute clinical concerns.

The parent will express some annoyance at being turned away from ED previously without any tests having been performed, but predominantly they will be upset and scared.

After 6 minutes ask the candidate to conclude the discussion and ask them to summarise the history, and to discuss their plan for investigations and management.

Ask them:
1. Please tell me what differential diagnoses you are considering, and why.
2. What would be your next steps in management?

Actor's instructions

You noticed bruising on Ben's arms and stomach this morning when he woke up. Ben is currently sleeping in your bed at night as he has been unwell with temperatures for the last two weeks, so you are certain he hasn't done anything to hurt himself in the night.

Ben is yours and your husband's only child; he was born at term, by a normal vaginal delivery, and has had no health problems to date. He sometimes picks up coughs and cold from other children at the childminder's, but usually gets over these illnesses quickly. You have been very worried as he has had a temperature of around 38°C almost every day for two weeks now, which is not normal for him – he also seems pale, and tired. He hasn't had a cough, cold, diarrhoea or vomiting, but you think he has lost his appetite and his clothes are definitely looser now. You have bought him to the Emergency Department twice in the last two weeks because of this but each time you were told he has a viral illness, to keep giving him regular paracetamol, and to bring him back if you were worried.

You are a freelance writer and work from home. You are happily married to Ben's father; the three of you live together. Ben's Dad is a lawyer and often works away from home, and has been abroad with work for the last two weeks. Normally Ben goes to a childminder three afternoons a week, but he has not been for the last two weeks due to the temperatures; no-one else has child caring duties. You are not known to social services and never have been. There is no medical family history of note – you and your husband have always been fit and well.

You aren't sure what is wrong with Ben, but he is really not himself and you are certain that this is something more than a viral infection. You are annoyed that you have been turned away from the Emergency Department twice already with no tests being done, but predominantly you are upset and scared something is seriously wrong.

HISTORY – NON-TRAUMATIC BRUISING

	Achieved	Not Achieved
Introduces self		
Clarifies who they are speaking to and relationship to child		
Elicits history of bruising from today		
Confirms that there is no history of trauma to explain bruising		
Elicits history of suspected weight loss		
Elicits history of recent temperature and ED visits with diagnosis of viral infection		
Performs systems review		
Clarifies Ben's past medical history		
Checks family history		
Enquires about social history, including who is at home		
Clarifies who has caregiving responsibility for Ben (parents, childminder)		
Asks about mother's ideas / concerns		
Responds appropriately to mother's concerns		
Summarises history and management plan concisely		
Considers sensible differential diagnosis		
Recognises patient requires discussion with senior		
Recognises need for blood tests; must mention FBC and blood film, may mention LDH/ESR/coagulation/CRP		
Recognises importance of examination (assessing for qualities of the bruises, hepatosplenomegaly, signs of anaemia, lymphadenopathy) +/- imaging (CXR to assess mediastinum, USS to assess spleen)		
Use appropriate lay terminology		
Non –judgemental approach		
Examiner's global mark	/5	
Actor's global mark	/5	
Total Station Mark	/30	

Learning Points

Apparently non-traumatic bruising has multiple potential causes; to help differentiate between them you must consider systems review to pick up subtle features in history. For example, a history of ongoing cough might increase the likelihood of a mycoplasma pneumonia with erythema multiforme (which can be mistaken for bruising by parents). A sensible differential diagnosis in this case would include:

1. A new oncological diagnosis, e.g. ALL
2. Non-accidental injury
3. Mycoplasma pneumonia with erythema multiforme
4. Henoch-Schönlein purpura
5. Meningococcal septicaemia

With any history of bruising, you must **always** consider non-accidental injury, even in situations where there are indications of an underlying organic cause. Ensure you have a full history of the time the bruising appeared – where was the child, what were they doing, who was caring for them, did they see the child injure themselves – as well as a full social history, including asking about social services involvement.

Whilst new oncological diagnoses are thankfully rare in children, Acute Lymphoblastic Leukaemia (ALL) is the most common childhood cancer, particularly in younger children. Even paediatricians in the smallest units will come across new cases each year, meaning you must know how it can present and what initial management steps are. Particularly, be aware that it often presents in an insidious manner (as in this case) as early signs and symptoms can mimic serial minor viral infections; if caught very early the FBC result may appear grossly normal, but abnormal cells will still be seen on blood film.

EXAMINATION STATIONS

16. EXAMINATION - ABDOMINAL EXAMINATION

Candidate's Instructions:

You are an FY1 doctor in the Paediatric Outpatient Clinic. You have just seen a 9 year old child with recurrent abdominal pain and the consultant asks you to perform a focused abdominal examination and present your findings.

With 2 minutes remaining the examiner will stop you, ask you to summarise back your findings and will ask you some direct questions.

Examiner's Instructions:

A 9 year old child has been referred by their GP to the Paediatric Outpatient Clinic with a 1 year history of recurrent central abdominal pain.

Abdominal examination is completely normal.

After 6 minutes ask the candidate to conclude the examination and ask them to summarise their findings, differential diagnosis, and to discuss their plan for investigations and management.

Actor's Instructions:

You are a 9 year old boy, who has recurrent abdominal pain. Examination findings are entirely normal throughout.

ABDOMINAL EXAMINATION OSCE

Task:	Achieved	Not Achieved
Introduces self		
Washes hands		
Clarifies who they are speaking to and relationship to child, gains consent for examination		
Conducts exam in systematic manner within a comfortable position and child appropriately exposed		
Inspect from end of bed		
Inspect hands		
Inspect conjunctivae		
Inspect mouth		
Expose abdomen with child lying flat and relaxed		
Inspects abdomen more closely		
Superficial palpation of all quadrants		
Deep palpation of all 4 quadrants		
Palpate for liver and spleen		
Palpate for kidneys		
Palpate hernial orifices		
Briefly inspect genitalia		
Auscultate for bowel sounds		
Ask to plot height and weight for child on a growth chart		
Summarises findings and presents succinctly		
Correctly suggests possible diagnoses of abdominal migraine, constipation, coeliac disease, functional abdominal pain		
Examiner's Global Mark	/5	
Actor / Helper's Global Mark	/5	
Total Station Mark	/30	

Learning Points

Abdominal pain is a common complaint in the Paediatric Outpatient Department. It is frequently benign and self-limiting, but careful history and examination are required to identify the small number of children presenting with serious organic disease. Many children will have simple constipation and this should be identified in the history and treated appropriately.

Symptoms associated with a higher prevalence of organic disease include: weight loss, bleeding (upper or lower GI tract), severe, persistent diarrhoea or vomiting, persistent right upper quadrant or right lower quadrant pain, fever, family history of inflammatory bowel disease, jaundice, urinary symptoms and abnormal examination findings.

Investigations are rarely useful in the absence of alarm symptoms, however coeliac disease can present with non-specific abdominal symptoms and should always be excluded with a coeliac screen.

17. EXAMINATION - NEWBORN EXAMINATION

Candidate's Instructions:

You are the FY1 doctor for Paediatrics and you have been asked to perform a routine newborn examination on a baby and present your findings back to your registrar. All the equipment that you need will be available on request.

With 2 minutes remaining the examiner will stop you, ask you to summarise back your findings and will ask you some direct questions.

Examiner's Instructions:

The candidate is a junior doctor on a post natal ward, and has been asked to perform a routine baby check on a well baby.

After 6 minutes ask the candidate to conclude the examination and ask them to summarise their findings, differential diagnosis, and to discuss their plan for investigations and management.

Ask them: 'Is there is any specific advice you would like to give the mother before she goes home?'

Actor's Instructions:

Examination findings are normal except for a soft systolic murmur heard at the upper right sternal edge. This does not radiate (if assessed), there is no heave or thrill (if assessed) and both femoral pulses are well felt. The baby is pink and not cyanosed.

If requested, tell the candidate that both pre and post ductal saturations are 98% in air and the mean four limb blood pressures are all within normal limits.

EXAMINATION - NEWBORN EXAMINATION

Task:	Achieved	Not Achieved
Introduces self		
Clarifies who they are speaking to and relationship to child, gets consent for examination		
Conducts newborn exam in systematic manner with baby in a comfortable position and appropriately exposed		
Feel fontanelle and sutures and measure head circumference (say will plot on growth chart)		
Assess facial features, inspect ears and neck		
Check red reflexes		
Visually inspect palate using tongue depressor and torch		
Auscultate chest for heart sounds and over lung fields		
Palpate femoral pulses		
Palpate abdomen to identify any masses or liver enlargement		
Examines hips (Barlow and Ortolani tests)		
Inspect hands and feet		
Inspect genitalia and anus (check for bilateral descent of testes in male)		
Inspect spine and sacrum		
Test moro reflex and assess tone in ventral suspension (baby should briefly bring head to horizontal plane)		
Comment on skin (birthmarks/rashes)		
Summarises findings and presents succinctly		
Correctly suggest checking pre and post ductal saturations		
Advises mother about signs of heart failure in a newborn		
Suggests plotting growth parameters on growth chart		
Examiner's Global Mark	/5	
Actor / Helper's Global Mark	/5	
Total Station Mark	/30	

Learning Points

Heart murmurs are common in first few days of life but are frequently innocent. Common causes include patent ductus arteriousus (PDA) (should close within 24 hours), flow murmurs and small septal defects such as patent foramen ovale (PFO), atrial septal defect (ASD) and ventricular septal defect (VSD) although the latter are commonly not heard until the child is a few weeks of age.

Babies with a murmur audible after 24 hours of life should be screened using pre and post ductal saturations (a difference of more than 2% is significant and warrants further investigation). Four limb blood pressures are often performed to help identify children with coarctation in which case the lower limb blood pressures will be more than 20 mmHg *lower* than the upper limb blood pressures which is the reverse of normal.

Parents in infants with heart murmurs should be advised of the signs of heart failure in a newborn. These include breathlessness, especially with feeding, sweatiness, lethargy, pallor and cyanosis.

18. EXAMINATION - RESPIRATORY EXAMINATION

Candidate's Instructions:

You are an FY1 doctor in Paediatrics. You have just seen a 15 year old boy with a chronic chest condition on the ward round and you have been asked to perform a respiratory examination and present your findings.

With 2 minutes remaining the examiner will stop you, ask you to summarise back your findings and will ask you some direct questions.

Examiner's Instructions:

A 15 year old boy with Cystic Fibrosis has been electively admitted to the ward for a course of intravenous antibiotics. He is currently well.

After 6 minutes ask the candidate to conclude the examination and ask them to summarise their findings, differential diagnosis, and to discuss their plan for investigations and management.

Ask 'In addition to the paediatrician, who else may be involved in this child's care?'.

Actor's Instructions:

You are a 15 year old boy with cystic fibrosis and are used to being examined by junior doctors for exams and in clinics. You are currently an inpatient for a planned course of antibiotics but are feeling well in yourself.

Respiratory examination reveals that he is short for his age, has clubbing of the fingernails and bibasal crackles, likely secondary to bronchiectasis. He also has an increased antero-posterior diameter of the chest.

EXAMINATION - RESPIRATORY EXAMINATION

Task:	Achieved	Not Achieved
Introduces self		
Clarifies who they are speaking to and relationship to child, gets consent for examination		
Washes hands		
Conducts exam in systematic manner within a comfortable position and child appropriately exposed		
Inspect from end of bed		
Note the presence of oxygen/inhalers/other medications at the bedside		
Inspect the hands (clubbing/cyanosis)		
Palpate radial pulse and count respiratory rate		
Looks for a BCG scar		
Inspect conjunctivae for pallor and tongue for central cyanosis		
Expose and inspect the chest		
Inspect chest from side during inspiration and expiration to look for increased antero-posterior diameter		
Palpate suprasternal notch for tracheal deviation		
Auscultate chest		
Percusses chest		
Palpates for tactile vocal fremitus		
Suggests plotting growth parameters on growth chart		
Ask to measure peak flow and oxygen saturations		
Summarises findings and presents succinctly		
Correctly suggests diagnosis of cystic fibrosis and identifies at least three people in MDT (doctor/nurse specialist/dietitian/physiotherapist/psychologist /pharmacist etc)		
Examiner's Global Mark	/5	
Actor / Helper's Global Mark	/5	
Total Station Mark	/30	

Learning Points

Cystic fibrosis is a genetic disease of exocrine gland function. There are numerous genetic mutations which give rise to the disease, the commonest in Northern Europe being the ΔF508 mutation which is present in up to 25% of cases. Abnormalities in chloride ion channel function lead to the production of thick, viscid secretions which have a number of effects.

Chronic production of mucus leads to airway plugging, inflammation and bronchiectasis as well as a pre-disposition to infection. Pancreatic exocrine function is affected, constipation is common and males are usually infertile. Patients can also have sinus involvement and eventually develop biliary obstruction and cirrhotic liver disease.

Management in a multi-disciplinary team is vital. Treatments for respiratory complications include regular chest physiotherapy and incentive spirometry, mucolytic drugs, regular prophylactic antibiotics and planned courses of intravenous antibiotics to prevent chest colonization and invasive infection. Pancreatic enzyme supplementation and dietetic support is necessary to achieve as near normal growth as possible and psychology input is important to help children adjust to living with a life-limiting disease.

19. EXAMINATION - UPPER LIMB NEUROLOGY

Candidate's Instructions:

You are an FY1 doctor in Paediatrics Paediatric Outpatient Department. A 9 year old girl presents with weakness in her arms. Your registrar has asked you to assess the motor neurology in the upper limbs of this patient and present your findings.

Examiner's Instructions:

A 9 year old girl has increased tone, weakness and hyperreflexia of the upper limbs bilaterally, and in all areas.

After 6 minutes ask the candidate to conclude the examination and ask them to summarise their findings, differential diagnosis, and to discuss their plan for investigations and management.

Ask them: "How they would you differentiate between an upper or lower motor neurone lesion."

Actor's Instructions:

You are a 9 year old girl who has weakness in your arms. At rest both arms are kept across your body, flexed at the elbows and wrists. Your arms are stiff in all muscle groups with clasp-knife responses at both elbows. You have increased deep tendon reflexes in all areas bilaterally. Power in all areas in reduced, with flexor muscles being stronger than extensor muscles.

EXAMINATION - UPPER LIMB NEUROLOGY

Task:	Achieved	Not Achieved
Introduces self		
Washes hands		
Clarifies who they are speaking to and relationship to child, gets consent for examination		
Appropriately exposes child		
Appropriately positions child		
Inspects patient from end of bed		
Inspect arms		
Assess tone in all muscle groups bilaterally		
Assess power in all muscle groups bilaterally (one arm at a time):		
Finger flexion (C8)		
Finger abduction (C8/T1)		
Wrist flexion/extension (C5/6)		
Elbow flexion(C5-6)/extension (C7/8)		
Abduction at shoulder (C5/6)		
Assess reflexes bilaterally (one arm at a time):		
Biceps (C5/6)		
Triceps (C6/7)		
Supinator (C5/6)		
Assess coordination (dysdiadochokinesis/past pointing/intention tremor)		
Summarises findings and presents succinctly		
Suggests upper motor neurone lesion		
Able to list differences between upper and lower motor neurone lesion findings		
Examiner's Global Mark	/5	
Actor / Helper's Global Mark	/5	
Total Station Mark	/30	

99

Learning Points

Remember to inspect the patient from the end of the bed. Taking note of the posture of the child's arms can reveal important features that will help your diagnosis. In this instance, the flexed posture of the arms are suggestive of increased muscle tone in an upper motor neurone lesion.

Remember to be gentle when examining a child with increased muscle tone. Sudden, forceful movements of stiff joints can be extremely painful and should be avoided. You may not need to fully extend the limb to establish that tone in increased!

Keep in mind the key differences in clinical findings that will help you differentiate upper and lower motor neurone lesions:

Upper Motor Neurone	Lower Motor Neurone
Flexed upper limb posture	Muscle wasting
Extended lower limb posture	Fasciculation
Increased tone	Reduced tone/flaccidity
Increased tendon reflexes	Reduced tendon reflexes

20. EXAMINATION - CARDIOVASCULAR EXAMINATION

Candidate's Instructions:

You are an FY1 doctor in Paediatrics. A 12 year old girl has been referred in by her GP for review as he noted a raised blood pressure (130/75) on examination in the surgery today. Your registrar asks you to examine her cardiovascular system and present your findings.

With 2 minutes remaining the examiner will stop you, ask you to summarise back your findings and will ask you some direct questions.

Examiner's Instructions:

A 12 year old girl has been referred by the GP with raised BP in the surgery today.

After 6 minutes ask the candidate to conclude the examination and ask them to summarise their findings, differential diagnosis, and to discuss their plan for investigations and management.

Actor's Instructions:

Cardiovascular examination reveals an ejection systolic murmur at the upper right sternal border which radiates to the interscapular area on the back. There is no heave or thrill palpable. Upper limb pulses are well felt. There is no radio-radial delay but radio femoral delay is present. Femoral pulses are more difficult to palpate but present.

If requested, four limb blood pressures are as follows:

RUL 135/70
LUL138/72
RLL 108/58
LLL 110/65

EXAMINATION - CARDIOVASCULAR

Task:	Achieved	Not Achieved
Introduces self		
Washes hands		
Clarifies who they are speaking to and relationship to child, gets consent for examination		
Conducts exam in systematic manner within a comfortable position and child appropriately exposed		
Inspects from end of bed		
Inspects hands & nails		
Palpate radial pulse (radio-radial and radio-femoral delay)		
Inspects conjunctivae		
Inspects mouth		
Exposes chest and inspects for surgical scars/chest wall deformity/hyperdynamic praecordium		
Palpate for heaves/thrills		
Auscultate in aortic, pulmonary, mitral and tricuspid areas		
Listens for radiation of ejection systolic murmur appropriately (to interscapular region for coarctation)		
Listen to lung bases		
Palpate liver		
Palpate femoral pulses (if not already done)		
Summarises findings and presents succinctly		
Correctly suggests possible diagnosis of aortic coarctation		
Suggests performing 4 limb BP measurement and able to identify abnormal results		
Suggests plotting growth parameters on growth chart		
Examiner's Global Mark	/5	
Actor / Helper's Global Mark	/5	
Total Station Mark	/30	

Learning Points

Coarctation of the aorta may present in the neonatal period when the ductus arteriosus closes and adequate systemic blood flow cannot be maintained. Babies present in shock with poor perfusion, tachycardia, absent femoral pulses and a difference in pre and post ductal saturations (pre-ductal higher than post-ductal). This is a medical emergency requiring immediate treatment with prostaglandin.

Many children with juxta-ductal coarctation (constriction distal to the origin of the left subclavian artery) are asymptomatic and do not present until late in childhood, often because of an incidental finding of a murmur (classically ejection systolic with radiation to back) or raised BP. Lower limb blood pressures will be lower than upper limb pressures (normally lower limbs should be higher than upper limbs). Radio-femoral delay may also be present on examination and is due to formation of collateral blood vessels that supply the distal aorta.

Coarctation is surgically corrected or can be dilated via cardiac catheterisation. Complications include re-coarctation and residual hypertension which can lead to intracranial haemorrhage or encephalopathy if severe.

21. EXAMINATION - CEREBELLAR EXAMINATION

Candidate's Instructions:

A 13 year girl old has presented to the ED with unsteadiness.

You are a FY1 in paediatric ED and you have been asked to perform a cerebellar examination and present your findings back to the paediatric team.

With 2 minutes remaining the examiner will stop you, ask you to summarise back your findings and will ask you some direct questions.

Examiner's Instructions:

A 13 year girl old has presented to the ED with unsteadiness.

The candidate is an F1 doctor in ED and they have been asked to perform a cerebellar examination and summarise their findings back to the team.

After 6 minutes ask the candidate to conclude the examination and ask them to summarise their findings, differential diagnosis, and to discuss their plan for investigations and management. Explore the differential diagnosis for cerebellar ataxia with the candidate.

Actor's Instructions:

A 13 year old girl has presented to the ED with unsteadiness. The candidate has been asked to perform a cerebellar examination.

Examination reveals a broad based gait. When walking heel-toe, you are off balance falling consistently to the right.

Romberg's test reveals unsteadiness to the right, and right sided pronator drift. The patient has slurred speech and struggle to say repetitive sounds, and difficulty in coordinating your right arm and leg with the finger-nose and heel-shin tests. There is evidence of dysdiadochokinesis on the right.

EXAMINATION - CEREBELLAR EXAMINATION

Task	Achieved	Not Achieved
Introduces self		
Washes hands		
Adequately exposes the child		
Examines general appearance of the child		
Tests posture: asks child to stand with feet together and eyes opened		
Romberg's test		
Inspects patient's gait		
Tests heel to toe gait		
Tests eye movements looking for nystagmus		
Test of staccato speech: "baby hippopotamus"		
Tests for pronator drift		
Tests for cerebellar rebound		
Tests tone in arms		
Tests for dysdiadochokinesis		
Tests for upper limb coordination: finger-to-nose test		
Tests tone in lower limbs		
Tests lower limb co-ordination: heel-to-shin test		
Suggests plotting growth parameters on growth chart		
Summarises findings to examiner		
Gives appropriate differential diagnosis		
Examiner's Global Mark	/5	
Actor / Helper's Global Mark	/5	
Total Station Mark	/30	

Learning Points

As with all examination in children it is important to take the child's age and development into consideration when examining the child. Consider their ability to walk, as they may be normally unsteady on their feet if still learning to walk. For co-ordination get them to reach out for toys or put bricks on top of each other.

DANISH is a good mnemonic to remember when performing the cerebellar examination. It stands for dysdiadochokinesis, ataxia, nystagmus, intention tremor, slurred speech and hypotonia. You should assess for all of these when performing your examination.

Causes of cerebellar ataxia include stroke, space-occupying lesions, head injury, infections both viral and bacterial, genetic causes such as Freidrich's & spinocerebellar ataxia. In children aged 2-10 years cerebellar ataxia can occur following viral illnesses. This can take up to 6 months to fully resolve.

22. EXAMINATION - CRANIAL NERVE EXAMINATION

Candidate's Instructions:

A 13 year old boy has been brought into the ED as parents are concerned that his smile is not equal since he woke up this morning.

You are the FY1 doctor in the paediatric team and have been asked to examine the child's cranial nerves and then summarise your findings back to the team.

With 2 minutes remaining the examiner will stop you, ask you to summarise back your findings and will ask you some direct questions.

Examiner's Instructions:

A 13 year old boy has been brought to the ED as parents are concerned his smile is not equal since he woke up this morning.

The FY1 doctor in the paediatric team has been asked to perform a cranial nerve examination and then summarise their findings back to the team. They do not need to perform a fundoscopy examination, Rinne and Weber tests or the gag reflex so please ask them to move on at these points.

After 6 minutes ask the candidate to conclude the examination and ask them to summarise their findings, differential diagnosis, and to discuss their plan for investigations and management.

Actor's Instructions:

You are a 13 year old boy who has attended ED as parents are concerned your smile has not been equal since you woke up this morning. The candidate who is an FY1 doctor has been asked to perform a cranial nerve examination on you.

Please follow all candidates' instructions; they should only be examining your head and neck.

The child's face is droopy on the right, with an unequal smile. He is unable to blow up his cheeks or raise his right eyebrow.

The remainder of the examination is normal.

EXAMINATION - CRANIAL NERVE EXAMINATION

Task:	Achieved	Not Achieved
Introduces self		
Washes hands		
Appropriate positioning of child		
General inspection of child		
Inspection of the face is it symmetrical, any swelling, are eyes both central		
Tests child's visual acuity (if old enough can they read a line of a book, or point out numbers)		
Tests visual fields by confrontation method		
Candidate indicates they would perform fundoscopy		
Examines eye movements		
Tests pupillary light reflexes and accommodation reflex		
Tests sensation in all three zones of trigeminal nerve		
Motor examination of face: clench teeth, open mouth against resistance, lift eyebrows, close eyes, blow out cheeks, show teeth, shrug shoulder and turn head to side against resistance		
Tests hearing in each ear		
Indicate would carry out Rinne and Weber tests		
Ask patient to say "ahh" and visualizes uvula deviation, asks patient to cough		
Ask patient to open mouth and stick out tongue and move to both sides		
Candidate indicates they would perform full neurological examination		
Suggests plotting growth parameters on growth chart		
Summarises findings to examiner		
Suggests appropriate differential diagnosis		
Examiner's Global Mark	/5	
Actor / Helper's Global Mark	/5	
Total Station Mark	/30	

Learning Points

Knowing the cranial nerve examination is important. Bell's palsy can be a common paediatric presentation. It is important to distinguish between this and other more sinister conditions. Bell's palsy is a paralysis of the muscles of facial expression supplied by the facial nerve (cranial nerve VII). It is possible to identify if it is an upper or lower motor neuron lesion. In an upper motor neuron lesion there is sparing of the forehead muscles due to alternative pathways being utilised. In lower motor neuron lesions the patient cannot wrinkle their forehead and may have difficulty closing their eye.

Not all children will be able to follow all instructions so it is important to adapt it to make it fun for the child whilst covering all areas. Think about using toys to test eye movements and visual fields. Asking them to point out letter and numbers instead of reading words and making the movements a bit of a game.

Take your time to learn the cranial nerves and their function; this will help when you are examining them.

Cranial Nerve	Motor or Sensory	Broad function
I - Olfactory	Sensory	Smell
II- Optic	Sensory	Vision
III- Oculomotor	Motor	Eye movements
IV - Trochlear	Motor	Superior oblique movement
V- Trigeminal	Both	Sensation to face and motor to muscles of mastication
VI- Abducens	Motor	Lateral rectus movement
VII- Facial	Both	Motor to muscles of facial expression, sensory to anterior 2/3 tongue
VIII – Vestibulo-ocular	Sensory	Hearing, balance
IX - Glossopharyngeal	Both	Swallow and gag reflex, taste posterior 1/3 tongue
X- Vagus	Both	Swallow and gag and speech
XI - Accessory	Motor	Shoulder and head movement
XII - Hypoglossal	Motor	Tongue movement, swallow and speech

23. EXAMINATION - EAR, NOSE AND THROAT EXAMINATION

Candidate's Instructions:

A 7 year girl old has presented to clinic with unilateral hearing loss for 1 week.

You are the FY1 in the Paediatric Outpatient Department and have been asked to perform an ear nose and throat examination and present your findings back to the consultant.

With 2 minutes remaining the examiner will stop you, ask you to summarise back your findings and will ask you some direct questions.

Examiner's Instructions:

A 7 year old girl has presented to clinic with unilateral hearing loss for 1 week.

The candidate is an FY1 doctor in the Paediatric Outpatient Department. They have been asked to perform an ear nose and throat examination and summarise their findings back to the consultant. The candidate should perform an ENT examination. They do not need to perform Rinne and Weber tests so please move them on at this stage.

After 6 minutes ask the candidate to conclude the examination and ask them to summarise their findings, differential diagnosis, and to discuss their plan for investigations and management.

Actor's Instructions:

You are a 7 year old girl who has presented to clinic with loss of hearing on the right side for about a week, but you have had no changes to your sense of smell.

When hearing is assessed, she is unable to hear quiet sounds on the right side, but are able to hear louder speech in the right ear when the left is occluded.

Nasal and mouth examination are normal.

EXAMINATION - EAR, NOSE AND THROAT EXAMINATION

Task:	Achieved	Not Achieved
Introduces self		
Washes hands		
Adequate exposure of the child		
Examines general appearance of the child		
Asks about patient's hearing		
Examines the external ear, pinna and behind the ear commenting on size, shape, any deformities		
Affixes appropriate size speculum to otoscope and uses appropriate technique when using the otoscope		
Examines ear canal commenting on wax, discharge, foreign bodies		
Examines tympanic membrane commenting on light reflex, effusions, perforations		
Assess patient's hearing		
Offers to do Rinne and Weber tests		
Examines the nose from the front, above and sides commenting on nasal discharge, scars, deformity		
Asks about sense of smell		
Examines the nose with an otoscope and thudicum speculum (if available)		
Examines the mouth and throat using otoscope and tongue depressor		
Does not cause the patient to gag when examining throat		
Palpates cervical and post auricular lymphnodes		
Summarise findings to examiner		
Suggests appropriate differential diagnosis		
Suggests plotting growth parameters on growth chart		
Examiner's Global Mark	/5	
Actor / Helper's Global Mark	/5	
Total Station Mark	/30	

Learning Points

ENT examination should be performed on all children presenting with a fever. Commonly throat and ear infections are the cause for the fever, and identifying these early can prevent further unnecessary investigations.

There is a wide differential for unilateral hearing loss and it is important to establish if it is conductive or sensorineural. In the older child Rinne and Weber tests will help. For unilateral conductive hearing loss consider as part of your differential; foreign body, glue ear, wax, perforation of the eardrum, infection, or previous surgery.

In young children always examine the throat last as the child is likely to become upset and further examination may be difficult. The optimal position for viewing a child's throat is with them on their parents' lap, their back against their parent's abdomen, with one of the parents' arms holding both the child's arm and the second holding their head. You may then use a tongue depressor to encourage them to open their mouth, although you may be asked not to do this in an exam setting.

24. EXAMINATION - LOWER LIMB NEUROLOGY

Candidate's Instructions:

An 8 year old boy who was born at 28 weeks gestation, who has a history of grade 3 IVH has been brought to clinic for his routine follow up.

You are an FY1 doctor in the Paediatric Outpatient clinic. You have been asked to examine the child's lower limb neurology and gait and then summarise your findings to your senior.

With 2 minutes remaining the examiner will stop you, ask you to summarise back your findings and will ask you some direct questions.

Examiner's Instructions:

An 8 year old boy who was born at 28 weeks gestation, with a history of grade 3 IVH has been brought to clinic for his routine follow up.

The candidate is an FY1 doctor in the clinic who has been asked to perform a lower limb neurological examination including assessment of gait then summarise their findings back to their senior. The candidate should perform the whole examination, please ask them to move on if they offer to test lower limb pain sensation.

After 6 minutes ask the candidate to conclude the examination and ask them to summarise their findings, differential diagnosis, and to discuss their plan for investigations and management.

It is most likely this scenario is pointing to a left hemiparesis following IVH. However, you can ask the candidate about other causes of hemiplegia. These will include stroke, head injury, brain tumour, infections, vasculitis, leukodystrophies.

Actor's Instructions:

You are an 8 year old boy who was born at 28 weeks gestation, who has a history of grade 3 IVH has been brought to clinic for his routine follow up.

The child displays a circumducting gait consistent with a left hemiplegia. There is increased tone throughout the left leg. Power is reduced in the knee flexors, with increased deep tendon reflexes in all areas in the left leg. Right leg examination is entirely normal. The candidate will not be asked to test pain sensation or proprioception.

EXAMINATION - LOWER LIMB NEUROLOGY

Task:	Achieved	Not Achieved
Introduces self		
Washes hands		
Adequate exposure of the child		
General inspection of child		
Inspects legs for muscle wasting or hypertrophy		
Examines child's gait: to walk in line, test heel toe gait, walking on tip toes and heels		
Ask candidate to stand up from sitting on floor		
Positions child appropriately on bed		
Examines tone		
Examines power in hips and knees		
Examines power in ankles and big toe		
Examines knee jerk and ankle jerk reflexes		
Examines plantar reflexes		
Examines child's co-ordination: heel-shin test		
Examines fine sensation in both legs		
Offers to test pain sensation and proprioception		
States they would complete the examination by examining the upper limbs and cranial nerves		
Suggests plotting growth parameters on growth chart		
Summarise findings to examiner		
Gives appropriate differential diagnosis		
Examiner's Global Mark	/5	
Actor / Helper's Global Mark	/5	
Total Station Mark	/30	

Learning Points

Not all children will be able to follow all instructions so it is important to adapt it to make it fun for the child whilst covering all areas. Think about using toys to test the child's coordination, or can they jump or hop. If they can't walk can they crawl. It may be difficult to get a child to relax in order to elicit the tendon reflexes, so consider using reinforcement techniques. Ask the child to clench their teeth at the same time you elicit the reflex, or ask them to clench their hands together.

The type of gait may indicate the underlying condition:

> Scissoring gait - spastic diplegia
> Waddling gait - muscular dystrophy.
> Antalgic gait -myositis or musculoskeletal pain
> Circumducting gait- hemiplegia

Be aware of the primitive reflexes and the age you would expect them to disappear.

Reflex	Onset	Disappears
Moro	Birth	2-3 months, may persist to 6 months
Rooting	Birth	4 months
Palmar grasp	Birth	5-6 months age
Plantar reflex	Birth	1 year
Tonic neck reflex	1 month	4 months

25. EXAMINATION - SKIN

Candidate's Instructions:

A 6 year old girl has presented to the Paediatric Outpatient Department with a rash that her parents feel is getting worse over the last three months over winter. The rash is seen in both antecubital fossae and to a lesser degree in both popliteal fossae. The rash is red in patches with dry and cracked areas too and the child is actively itching them.

You are an FY1 doctor in the clinic and have been asked to examine the child's skin and then summarise your findings to your senior.

With 2 minutes remaining the examiner will stop you, ask you to summarise back your findings and will ask you some direct questions.

Examiner's Instructions:

A 6 year old girl has presented to the Paediatric Outpatient Department with a rash that her parents feel is getting worse over the last three months over winter. The rash is seen in both antecubital fossae and to a lesser degree in both popliteal fossae. The rash is red in patches with dry and cracked areas too and the child is actively itching them.

The candidate is an FY1 doctor in the clinic who has been asked to perform an examination of the skin and summarise their findings back to their senior.

After 6 minutes ask the candidate to conclude the examination and ask them to summarise their findings, differential diagnosis, and to discuss their plan for investigations and management.

Actor's Instructions:

A 6 year old girl has presented to the Paediatric Outpatient Department with a rash that her parents feel is getting worse over the last three months over winter. The rash is seen in both antecubital fossae and to a lesser degree in both popliteal fossae. The rash is red in patches with dry and cracked areas too and the child is actively itching them.

The candidate has been asked to perform an examination of the skin.

At 6 minutes they will be asked to summarise their findings to the examiner.

EXAMINATION - SKIN

Task:	Achieved	Not Achieved
Introduces self		
Washes hands		
Ensures light is adequate for examination		
Examines general appearance of the child		
Adequately exposes the child		
Describes distribution of skin lesions		
Describes of colour of the lesion		
Describes shape of the lesion		
Measures the lesion with tape measure		
Ensures there is no pain over lesions		
Gently palpates any skin lesions		
Examines finger and toe nails		
Examines hair and scalp		
Examines mucous membranes		
Examines for lymphadenopathy		
States would examine skin using Woods lamp		
Uses appropriate dermatological terms to describe lesion		
Suggests plotting growth parameters on growth chart		
Summarises findings to examiner		
Suggests appropriate differential diagnosis		
Examiner's Global Mark	/5	
Actor / Helper's Global Mark	/5	
Total Station Mark	/30	

Learning Points

Be able to describe skin lesions using dermatological terms

Macule	Area of colour change less than 1.5cm diameter
Patch	Large area of colour change bigger than a macule, with flat surface
Papule	Small palpable lesion less than 0.5cm in diameter.
Nodule	Enlargement of a papule
Cyst	Fluid filled nodule or papule
Plaque	Raised flat topped lesion greater than a papule
Vesicle	Fluid filled blister, less than 0.5cm
Bulla	Large fluid filled blister
Secondary skin lesions	
Scaling	Increase in dead cells on surface of the skin
Lichenification	Palpably thickened skin
Crusting	Pus exuding through eroded epidermis
Excoriation	Scratch mark
Ulceration	Sore on skin

Know the common skin conditions that affect children including and not exclusive to:

Eczema, pityriasis rosea, chickenpox, impetigo, warts, hand- foot and mouth disease, scarlet fever, tinea, measles, molluscum contagiosum, psoriasis, urticaria

When examining a child always be careful to expose all areas, rashes can hide in the axilla, behind the ears or on the buttocks. However, it is important to keep the child warm whilst doing this.

EXPLANATION STATIONS

26. COMMUNICATION - EXPLAIN ASTHMA TO AN OLDER CHILD

Candidate's Instructions:

Sarah is 14 and she has recently been diagnosed with asthma. You are the FY1 on the ward and your Consultant has asked you to explain to Sarah what asthma is and why she needs to take inhalers. They had a brief chat about asthma on the ward round this morning, but a more detailed explanation is required before Sarah goes home. You should explain to Sarah what asthma is and that she will need preventer and reliever inhalers after discharge from hospital. As part of your explanation, you should ensure that Sarah knows when to seek advice from an adult.

You see Sarah on the ward with her Mum before she goes home.

With 2 minutes remaining the examiner will stop you, ask you to summarise back your findings and will ask you some direct questions.

Examiner's Instructions:

Sarah is a 14-year-old girl and has recently been diagnosed with asthma, following an admission to the children's ward with a wheezy episode. She is now well and ready for discharge home.

The FY1 has been asked to explain to Sarah what asthma is, including the lifelong nature of the condition. The candidate should use age appropriate language to explain asthma to Sarah. They should enquire about triggers and ensure Sarah knows when to take medication and seek advice from an adult if she is unwell.

At 6 minutes, stop the candidate and ask them if there is anything further they wish to add.

Actor's Instructions:

You are Sarah, a 14-year-old girl who has been diagnosed with asthma. You have been told a little bit about what asthma is and understand that it is a condition where the airways in the lungs tighten, making it difficult to breathe. This causes you to have a cough and a tight feeling in your chest, as well as a wheeze. It is usually triggered when you exercise. You know you have to take inhalers but you are not really sure how long for. You are a bit worried about school and what you need to do if you feel unwell or need your inhalers at school.

You want to understand what asthma is, why you need your inhalers and when you need to talk to and adult about your condition, before you go home.

If any medical language is used or there are words that you don't understand, you should ask the candidate to explain what is meant.

You are on the ward with your Mum when the doctor comes to talk to you.

COMMUNICATION - EXPLAIN ASTHMA TO AN OLDER CHILD

Task:	Achieved	Not Achieved
Introduces self to young person and parent		
Clarifies who they are speaking to and relationship to child/young person		
Explains that they have come to talk about the condition with young person and parent		
Asks the young person if anyone has spoken to them before about their condition		
Asks the young person what their current understanding asthma is		
Explains what asthma is in simple terms		
Asks about triggers for symptoms		
Explains that inhaler medication will improve symptoms		
Explains that the condition is lifelong and will require preventer medication to keep well		
Explains what different inhalers are for		
Advises to seek adult help If feeling very unwell and out of breath		
Advises to seek adult help if using reliever medication very frequently or more frequently than usual		
Main focus of communication is with the young person and not the parent.		
Explains underlying condition, and avoids use of medical terms or jargon		
If any medical terms used, explains what they mean		
Uses age appropriate language		
Summarises discussion concisely		
Clarifies understanding of explanation that has been given		
Asks if the child or parent has any further questions		
Offers information leaflet		
Examiner's Global Mark	/5	
Actor / Helper's Global Mark	/5	
Total Station Mark	/30	

Learning Points

Clarify with both young person what explanations may or may not have been given previously, and allow the young person to explain in their own words what they understand already.

Communication should be with the young person and not their parent. Asthma is being explained to the teenager, for them to understand. Use age appropriate language and not medical terms or words that may not be fully understood.

Ensure the young person knows when to seek advice from an adult as although they may be independently managing their condition on a day-to day basis, they need to be certain about when to seek help in order to avoid an undetected deterioration in their condition.

27. COMMUNICATION - EXPLAIN VENEPUNCTURE TO A CHILD

Candidate's Instructions:

Nathan is 6 and has come to the Paediatric Outpatient Department for a blood test, as part of investigations for recurrent abdominal pain. He has never had a blood test before. You are the FY1 doctor working in outpatients today and have been asked to apply the local anaesthetic cream to his skin, 30 minutes before his appointment and explain to him what will happen when he has his blood test. Nathan is accompanied by his mother.

Examiner's Instructions:

Nathan is 6 and has come to the Paediatric Outpatient Department for a blood test, as part of investigations for recurrent abdominal pain. He has never had a blood test before. The FY1 doctor working in outpatients today has been asked to apply the local anaesthetic cream to Nathan's skin 30 minutes before the appointment and explain what the blood test entails. Nathan is accompanied by his mother.

Actor's Instructions:

1. You are 6 years old and have come to the hospital for a blood test. You have never had one before and you are frightened that it will really hurt. You know that a needle is used to take the blood as your friend told you that when you have a blood test a really huge needle is stuck in your arm. You don't want to have a blood test and you don't think there is anything the doctor can say that will change your mind. You are definitely going to ask if it will hurt.

2. You are Nathan's mother. You have brought him for a blood test to try and work out why he keeps having episodes of abdominal pain. He is frightened about the blood test and although you have tried to explain to him what will happen, you have only had one blood test yourself and you think it might be different for children.

If the doctor manages to explain to you and your son what will happen in words that he understands, you think he will sit still and have the blood test. If Nathan doesn't understand what will happen or thinks the blood test will hurt a lot, then it is likely that he will get very upset and refuse to allow the blood test to be performed.

COMMUNICATION - EXPLAIN VENEPUNCTURE TO A CHILD

Task:	Achieved	Not Achieved
Introduces self		
Clarifies who they are speaking to and relationship to child		
Build rapport with child and parent		
Clarifies child's and parent's current understanding of blood test and reason for it		
Explains the reason for the blood test in broad terms		
States that parent can stay with child throughout		
Explains that the cream for the skin makes it numb and should stop it hurting but it		
Child may still feel some discomfort		
Clearly states that the blood test will be done		
Explains that the child will need to sit still		
Explains the skin will be cleaned and that this may feel cold		
States the procedure may take a few minutes		
Uses age appropriate language and explains any medical terms used		
Offers distraction (e.g with book, DVD) or involvement of play therapist		
Suggest demonstration of the blood test with a toy		
Explains who will perform the procedure		
Reassures child that his mother can stay in the room with him for the procedure		
Is not untruthful and/or and tell the child that the procedure is completely painless		
Does not suggest that child may be physically restrained if unwilling for blood test		
Has calm and empathetic approach		
Examiner's Global Mark	/5	
Actor / Helper's Global Mark	/5	
Total Station Mark	/30	

Learning Points

It is best to explain to the child calmly what you are going to do. Give them choices about where they sit and what distraction they would like. Play specialists play a huge role in this and early involvement is key to gain the optimal result for the patient.

Never lie – if a procedure is going to hurt then say so, but tell the child what will be done to minimise this.

It often helps to show the child what will happen, using the same equipment and a toy doll or teddy bear.

28. COMMUNICATION - EXPLAIN ASTHMA TO PARENT OF A YOUNG CHILD

Candidate's Instructions:

Sarah is 8 and she has recently been diagnosed with asthma. You are the FY1 on the ward and your Consultant has asked you if you will explain to Sarah's parents what asthma is and why she needs to take her blue inhaler if she feels wheezy. Sarah is on the ward with her Father and they are about to be discharged home, following an admission with a wheezy episode.

They have been shown how to use the inhaler whilst on the ward (you are **not** expected to teach inhaler technique) and Sarah's father has asked of he can speak with a doctor about her condition and her medication before going home.

With 2 minutes remaining the examiner will stop you, ask you to summarise back your findings and will ask you some direct questions.

Examiner's Instructions:

Sarah is an 8-year-old girl and has recently been diagnosed with asthma, following an admission to the children's ward with a wheezy episode. She is now well and ready for discharge home.

The FY1 has been asked to explain to Sarah's Father what asthma is and why Sarah will need to take an inhaler if she feels wheezy. The family has been shown how to use an inhaler whilst on the ward and the candidate is not expected to teach inhaler technique. Sarah's father has requested to speak to a doctor about asthma and the medication needed, before they leave the ward.

At 6 minutes, stop the candidate and ask them if there is anything further they wish to add.

Actor's Instructions:

You are the father of Sarah, an 8-year-old girl who has been diagnosed with asthma. The ward doctor has come to explain to you what asthma is and why Sarah will need to use an inhaler if she feels wheezy.

Sarah has recently been admitted to the ward with a wheezy episode that seemed to start when she was doing PE at school. You have noticed that she often seems much more out of breath than her friends when she is running around and wonder if this is related.

You have asked the Consultant who saw you on the ward this morning if there is someone available to explain Sarah's condition and her medication, before you go home. You have been shown how to use the inhaler by the nursing staff on the ward. You have been told when to use it but remain unsure about what to do when you leave hospital.

If any medical language is used and the candidate does not explain what they mean, you may ask them to clarify.

COMMUNICATION - EXPLAIN ASTHMA TO PARENT OF A YOUNG CHILD

Task:	Achieved	Not Achieved
Introduces self to both child and parent		
Clarifies who they are speaking to and relationship to child		
Explains that they have come to talk about the condition with child and parent		
Asks if any explanation has been given previously		
Asks the parent to explain what their understanding of asthma is		
Explains asthma physiology in simple terms to child and parent		
Uses appropriate language, avoiding medical jargon		
If any medical terms used, explains what they mean		
Explains common symptoms of asthma (e.g cough, tight feeling in chest, difficulty in breathing)		
Explains common signs to look for (e.g audible wheeze, signs of respiratory distress)		
Asks about triggers for symptoms		
Explains that inhaler medication will improve symptoms		
Ensures parent clear about when to use medication		
Suggests use of inhaler prior to exercise		
Asks if parent knows how to give medication		
Ensures parent knows to seek medical advice in the event of acute deterioration		
Ensures parent knows to seek medical advice if child using reliever medication more than usual		
Clarifies understanding of explanation that has been given		
Summarises consultation		
Asks if the child or parent has any further questions		
Examiner's Global Mark	/5	
Actor / Helper's Global Mark	/5	
Total Station Mark	/30	

Learning Points

Clarify with both child and parent what explanations may or may not have been given previously. Allow the child to explain in their own words what they understand.

Use age appropriate language and not medical terms or words that a young child will not understand. Explain what any medical jargon means in simple terms.

When the child is present, communication should be with the child and not their parent. Asthma is being explained to the child, for them to understand. You may have to answer additional questions from the parent, but the focus of the communication should be with the child, in a way that they understand.

29. COMMUNICATION - EXPLAIN A FEBRILE SEIZURE TO A PARENT

Candidate's Instructions:

Ben is 18 months old. He was admitted to the children's ward following a febrile convulsion. He had a runny nose and temperature for 3 days before the convulsion. His fever was 39.2C at the time. It lasted 3 minutes and his mother described shaking of both his arms and his legs and Ben was not responding to her. It stopped by itself before the ambulance arrived and Ben has been very well since admission to the ward. You are the FY1 doctor on the ward and have been asked to explain to Ben's mother exactly what a febrile convulsion is.

With 2 minutes remaining the examiner will stop you, ask you to summarise back your findings and will ask you some direct questions.

Examiner's Instructions:

Ben is 18 months old. He was admitted to the children's ward following a febrile convulsion. He had a runny nose and temperature for 3 days before the convulsion. His fever was 39.2C at the time. It lasted 3 minutes and his mother described shaking of both his arms and his legs and Ben was not responding to her. It stopped by itself before the ambulance arrived and Ben has been very well since admission to the ward.

The FY1 doctor has been asked to explain to Ben's mother exactly what a febrile convulsion is. The candidate should give an explanation to the parent, elicit any concerns they have and deal with any queries appropriately.

At 6 minutes, stop the candidate and ask them if there is any further advice they wish to give Ben's parents.

Actor's Instructions:

Your son Ben is 18 months old and he has been admitted to the children's ward following a febrile convulsion. He had been unwell at home with a fever and runny nose for three days and then had a high fever of over 39°C at home. He became unresponsive and began shaking and jerking both his arms and legs. You were extremely worried and called an ambulance. The movements had stopped by the time the ambulance arrived and Ben did seem better in himself but he was still sleepy. Since you arrived at the hospital, he has been moved to the ward and although he is back to his usual self now, you still aren't quite sure what happened. You remember the ambulance crew mentioning something about a "fit" but were so worried at the time that you didn't really take much in. You have asked for someone to come and explain to you what happened.

You have a friend who has a little girl with epilepsy and she has seizures very frequently. You want to know that if Ben has also had a fit or seizure, then does he have epilepsy too and will he need to have medication or have fits again?

COMMUNICATION - EXPLAIN A FEBRILE SEIZURE TO A PARENT

Task:	Achieved	Not Achieved
Introduces self to parent		
Clarifies who they are speaking to and relationship to child		
Explains that they have come to talk about the reason for admission to the hospital		
Asks if any explanation has been given previously by other members of staff		
Asks the parent to explain what their understanding is of the febrile convulsion		
Explains a febrile seizure is a fit/seizure caused by a fever		
Explains it is caused by a sudden increase in body temperature		
Explains fever itself is not harmful but a sign the body is fighting infection		
Explains it is common in young children		
Explains febrile seizure is most common between 6 months and 6 years		
Explains most children will only have 1 febrile convulsion but some do have them again at times of high fever		
Clarifies that with simple febrile convulsions, there is no increase in risk of epilepsy		
Reassures parent the febrile convulsion is not harmful to the child (e.g not associated with brain damage)		
Explains common signs of a convulsion		
Explains what to do if Ben has a further convulsion (stay calm, place child on side, call ambulance)		
Appropriate use of language with explanation of any medical terms used		
Clarifies understanding of explanation that has been given		
Summarises consultation		
Asks if the child or parent has any further questions		
Offers information leaflet		
Examiner's Global Mark	/5	
Actor / Helper's Global Mark	/5	
Total Station Mark	/30	

Learning Points

Febrile convulsions can be very frightening for parents to witness, so it is important to have an empathetic approach, and acknowledge and address their questions.

There is often concern that febrile convulsions will lead to epilepsy and it is important that you explain this is not the case, as this is often a major cause of anxiety.

Ensure you explain to parents what to do should it happen again. This should include removing objects that a child may injure themselves on in the middle of a seizure, and simple advice regarding not overheating or rapidly cooling a child who is likely to have a fever. Most ED departments have an information leaflet that can be given to people to take home for reference.

30. COMMUNICATION – DISCUSS USE OF ANTIBIOTICS IN A VIRAL ILLNESS

Candidate's Instructions:

Jack is 18 months old and has been diagnosed with a viral upper respiratory tract infection. He attended the Emergency Department with a 24-hour history of a runny nose, dry cough and a fever. He is generally well in himself, eating and drinking as usual and playing in the waiting room. His mother wants him to have antibiotics for his infection but these have not been prescribed. You are the FY1 doctor in ED and have been asked to talk to Jack's mother.

Examiner's Instructions:

Jack is 18 months old and has been diagnosed with a viral upper respiratory tract infection. He attended the ED with a 24-hour history of a runny nose, dry cough and a fever. He is generally well in himself, eating and drinking as usual and playing in the waiting room. His mother wants him to have antibiotics for his infection but these have not been prescribed. The FY1 doctor has been asked to talk to her by the ED nursing staff.

Actor's Instructions:

You are the mother of Jack, who is 18 months old. You have asked to speak with a doctor.

You have brought Jack to the Paediatric Emergency Department as he has had a dry cough, runny nose and a high fever for 24 hours. The doctor who assessed Jack said that he had a viral infection and advised you to give paracetamol if needed. You are concerned that Jack has a chest infection and should have antibiotics. You have an older child who was admitted to hospital with a chest infection when he was a similar age to Jack. He received antibiotics and you want Jack to have the same treatment.

It is 2am and you have had very little sleep in the past 24 hours, as Jack has been miserable and coughing constantly. You want the antibiotics so that Jack will get better. You do not wish for him to need admission to hospital, as your older child did.

If the doctor is unable to explain to you why Jack has not been given antibiotics, you become frustrated and ask to speak with a more senior doctor.

If the explanation is satisfactory, you are reassured and willing to take Jack home.

COMMUNICATION – DISCUSS USE OF ANTIBIOTICS IN A VIRAL ILLNESS

Task:	Achieved	Not Achieved
Introduces self		
Clarifies who they are speaking to and relationship to child		
Seeks clarification about what has been explained so far		
Elicits parents understanding of the role of antibiotics		
Elicits parental concerns		
Elicits brief history of viral symptoms		
Explains that antibiotics not effective in treatment of viral infection		
Explains risk of side effects of antibiotics when used inappropriately: diarrhoea, resistance		
Explains usual course of viral infections		
Ensures parent satisfied with explanation of viral infection		
Asks if the parent has any further questions		
Empathetic approach to parent		
Uses appropriate language		
Explains any medical terms used		
Offers to discuss with senior if needed		
Does not offer antibiotics as treatment for the viral infection		
Summarises consultation		
Advises parent to return for review if child deteriorates or does not improve		
Offers information leaflet		
Non-judgemental approach		
Examiner's Global Mark	/5	
Actor / Helper's Global Mark	/5	
Total Station Mark	/30	

Learning Points

When providing additional information to a patient/parent who has been seen by another professional, you should always clarify what has already been explained in order to minimize any misunderstanding or miscommunication.

Do not dismiss the concerns of a patient or parent, however unfounded you may feel they are. They often have good reasons that you may be unaware of unless you explore the situation in more detail.

Antibiotics are not effective in the treatment of viral infections and should not be prescribed. Viral infections require symptomatic treatment only and will resolve with time. As differentiating between a bacterial and viral infection can be clinically challenging, the child should be brought back for re-evaluation if symptoms are worsening or not settling. This is termed "safety netting".

31. COMMUNICATION – COUNSELLING FOR IMPENDING PRETERM DELIVERY

Candidate's Instructions:

A woman who is 25 weeks pregnant has been admitted to Labour ward with contractions. On examination her cervix is found to be 5cm dilated and the obstetric team expect her to deliver in the next few hours. This is her first pregnancy and except for being treated for a UTI 1 week ago there has been nothing else untoward during the antenatal period.

You are a junior doctor in the paediatric team and have been asked to speak to the mother about her impending premature delivery.

With 2 minutes remaining the examiner will stop you, ask you to summarise back your findings and will ask you some direct questions.

Examiner's Instructions:

A woman at 25 weeks gestation has been brought to Labour Ward with contractions and cervical dilatation. She is expected to deliver in the next few hours.

The junior doctor in the paediatric team has been asked to speak to the mother about the impending preterm delivery.

At 6 minutes, stop the candidate and ask them if there is any further advice they wish to give.

Actor's Instructions:

You are 25 weeks pregnant to your first baby and unexpectedly have developed contractions. The obstetric team have told you that the baby may be delivered in the next few hours and gave you an injection of steroids to help with the baby's lungs. You are extremely anxious and scared.

Prior to this, your pregnancy so far has been going very well with normal scans and blood tests. You had a water infection one week ago that was treated with antibiotics. Following meetings with your midwife you had made a plan for a natural home birth and you are very keen to exclusively breastfeed your baby. You wonder if you can still do this if the baby is born prematurely. You also want to know if there is anything to be done to prevent the baby from being delivered early.

Other question that cross your mind is whether the prematurity will affect the baby's brain and development. You become upset when the subject of death or disability is discussed. Your partner is currently in the United States on a business trip and you have been on your own at home. However, your parents live close by and you would like the doctor to come back and explain things again when they arrive.

COMMUNICATION – COUNSELLING FOR IMPENDING PRETERM DELIVERY

Task:	Achieved	Not Achieved
Introduces self		
Clarifies who they are speaking to		
Sets the agenda and explain purpose of discussion		
Establishes current understanding of preterm birth and consequences for babies		
Explains that premature baby is unable to survive without support and may need resuscitation		
Explains that paediatric team will be present at delivery		
Explains that baby will be assessed and supported with breathing and circulation as required		
Explains that baby will be shown to mother and admitted to neonatal unit for treatment		
Explains that prematurity is directly linked with morbidity and mortality		
Explains that baby will need breathing support either by intubation or non-invasive methods		
Explains that baby will have brain scans and development will be monitored long term		
Explains that baby will initially be unable to feed independently and will need TPN		
Emphasises importance of breast milk as protector against gut disease and encourages mother to express		
Explains that baby will need surveillance eg ROP screen to identify and address problems early		
Reassure mother that all steps will be taken to optimise outcome for the baby once born		
Asks parent if they have any further questions		
Summarises consultation & actions from here on		
Offers to come back to speak to the mother again later if she wishes		
Uses appropriate language and explains medical jargon		
Offers information leaflet		
Examiner's Global Mark	/5	
Actor / Helper's Global Mark	/5	
Total Station Mark	/30	

Learning Points

Care of the preterm infant is a developing field as new evidence becomes available that helps tailor interventions and optimises outcome.

Morbidity and mortality rates are directly linked to the degree of prematurity in infants. The EPICure series of studies of survival and later health among babies and young people who were born at extremely low gestations offers data than can be useful when discussing prognosis with parents (EPICure 2006)

In addition to long term outcomes it is also important to discuss the process of resuscitation. Most parents do not expect the interventions and resuscitation performed during the delivery of an extremely premature infant and can find the experience quite traumatic. Briefing them before the delivery on what is going to happen helps them cope with this better.

32. COMMUNICATION – CONCERNS REGARDING ROUTINE IMMUNISATION

Candidate's Instructions:

A 2 month old boy is due to have his first lot of immunisations. He has arrived at a Community Paediatric clinic with his mother who has done some reading online about immunisations and would like to discuss her concerns with the medical team.

You are the FY1 doctor in the paediatric team and have been asked to speak to the mother about routine immunisations.

With 2 minutes remaining the examiner will stop you, ask you to summarise back your findings and will ask you some direct questions.

Examiner's Instructions:

A 2 month old child has arrived for his first lot of routine immunisations. The mother has done some online research about immunisations and has some concerns.

The FY1 doctor in the paediatric team has been asked to address these concerns and explain the indications and side effects of routine immunisations.

At 6 minutes, ask the candidate to conclude the discussion and ask them to name the conditions covered by the first set of immunisations.

Actor's Instructions:

Your 2 month old baby is due to have his first immunisations and you have been doing some research online about them. You have found lots of conflicting information with some websites (e.g. the NHS website) recommending them while others warning against them. You are particularly concerned about claims that immunisations can cause allergic reactions and that they are linked with autism.

Your baby is a first child born following a natural delivery and has been doing very well so far. He is exclusively breastfed and has never been ill. You are worried that the immunisations might hurt him and may also lead him to develop a fever. You would like to know what the risks would be if you do not have him immunised.

If you feel that the doctor has listened to your concerns and has addressed all of your fears about immunizations explaining all the risks and benefits you would be happy to proceed with the immunizations. However, if you feel that your concerns have been dismissed without proper explanations do ask for some more time to think about it before you agree for immunizations to be given.

COMMUNICATION – CONCERNS REGARDING ROUTINE IMMUNISATION

Task:	Achieved	Not Achieved
Introduces self		
Clarifies who they are speaking to and relationship to child		
Sets the agenda and explain purpose of discussion		
Clarifies parental concerns		
Establishes current understanding of immunisation		
Outlines immunisation schedule including rotavirus oral vaccine		
Highlights benefits of immunisations including protection from potentially fatal conditions		
Highlights benefits of herd immunity		
Explains that anaphylaxis is a serious but very rare complications of immunisation		
Briefly mentions how to spot an allergic reaction to immunisation and what to do.		
Explains possibility of self limiting coryzal symptoms after immunisation.		
Explains that pain and erythema can be expected around site of injection for brief period		
Encourages use of paracetamol for above symptoms		
Reassures mother that there is no proven link between immunisations and autism		
Emphasises the importance of consulting reliable sources for medical information eg NHS website		
Asks parent if they have any further questions		
Summarises consultation & actions from here on		
Non-judgemental approach		
Uses appropriate language & explains any jargon used		
Offers information leaflet		
Examiner's Global Mark	/5	
Actor / Helper's Global Mark	/5	
Total Station Mark	/30	

Learning Points

It is important to know the recent schedule of routine immunisations and the conditions each of those protects against. Recently immunisations against Rotavirus, Meningitis B, Flu virus and Human Papillomavirus (HPV)have been added to the routine schedule in the UK.

There are very few contraindications to routine vaccination for children: these include specific allergies to the vaccine or its components and immunosuppression in the case of live vaccines.

Online resources such as the NHS Choices website and Patient.co.uk offer reliable information for parents about immunisations. This can help reinforce verbal information and help distinguish from misleading information widely available that is not evidence based. Giving patients leaflets to take away and digest and then follow up with their own GP is often the best strategy.

33. COMMUNICATION – EXPLAIN NEED FOR TRANSFER TO TERTIARY UNIT FOR ACUTE CONDITION

Candidate's Instructions:

A newborn baby boy was born in poor condition following shoulder dystocia. He has been intubated and ventilated due to low Apgar scores. Blood gases have been borderline and for the first two hours the baby was doing well but then was noted to be having focal seizures. The baby was given phenobarbitone and the seizures stopped. However, in view of this it is decided to transfer the baby to a tertiary centre for therapeutic hypothermia and further investigations.

You are the junior doctor in the paediatric team and have been asked to speak to the family to explain the change in his condition and need to transfer the baby to a tertiary centre for ongoing care.

With 2 minutes remaining the examiner will, ask you to summarise back your findings and will ask you some direct questions.

Examiner's Instructions:

A newborn baby has been delivered in poor condition following shoulder dystocia and there is evidence of hypoxic ischaemic encephalopathy. Two hours after birth the baby had seizures which indicated the need to start therapeutic hypothermia and transfer the baby to a tertiary centre for ongoing management.

The junior doctor in the paediatric team has been asked to speak to the parents to explain the need for transfer to a tertiary centre.

At 6 minutes, ask the candidate to conclude the discussion and ask them how they would differentiate between mild, moderate and severe hypoxic ischaemic encephalopathy in the newborn from initial clinical examination.

Actor's Instructions:

Your baby was born quite unwell a few hours ago totally unexpectedly. You had a normal pregnancy but the midwives told you that the baby's shoulder got stuck during delivery. Instead of giving the baby to you after birth he was taken away to the paediatricians and was admitted to the special baby unit where he is now breathing with the help of a machine. You visited the baby earlier and you were told that the baby was stable and hopefully the tube would be removed soon. You are shocked and upset when you hear that he has had seizures and needs to be moved to a different hospital.

You are very worried about the long term implications of what has happened and specifically if the baby has suffered brain damage. You are distressed about not having the baby with you and not being able to breastfeed. You are worried that he will be far away and you will not be able to see him. You are reassured when you are told that you may visit him at any time.

You hope that he recovers quickly and that you are able to take him home soon. However, you are happy to agree with any medical treatment that is considered best for him as long as it is properly explained.

COMMUNICATION – EXPLAIN NEED FOR TRANSFER TO TERTIARY UNIT FOR ACUTE CONDITION

Task:	Achieved	Not Achieved
Introduces self		
Clarifies who they are speaking to and relationship to child, ask for child's name		
Sets the agenda and explain purpose of discussion		
Clarifies parent's understanding of events so far		
Reiterates that baby was deprived of oxygen at birth which is the cause of its current condition		
Explain that baby had a seizure that was treated with medication and baby is now stable		
Explain that seizure shows that brain has been affected and treatment is needed to protect it from further damage		
Explain that cooling treatment can be given at a tertiary centre but passive cooling already started		
Explain that baby will be transferred safely by the transport team		
Explain that further tests eg MRI and EEG will be performed to better define prognosis		
Explain that it is too soon to determine prognosis but all steps are taken to optimise it		
Explain that length of stay at tertiary centre will depend on baby's progress.		
Explain baby will be nil by mouth for now but milk can be expressed and given to baby later.		
Explain that long term surveillance will be required		
Explain that 24 hour access to the baby will be facilitated for the parents by receiving hospital		
Asks parent if they have any further questions		
Summarises consultation & actions from here on		
Offers to come back and update parents again later		
Uses appropriate language & explains any jargon		
Offers information leaflet		
Examiner's Global Mark	/5	
Actor / Helper's Global Mark	/5	
Total Station Mark	/30	

Learning Points

In developed countries, hypoxic ischaemic encephalopathy (HIE) affects 3–5 infants per 1000 live births, and is an important cause of cerebral palsy and developmental difficulties. Diagnosis and severity of HIE can be determined using the Sarnat & Sarnat staging method (Sarnat & Sarnat 1976).

Whilst damage from the primary insult cannot be repaired, moderate cooling of the body (to between 32 and 34 degrees Celsius) has been shown to prevent further brain damage and death in asphyxiated newborn infants, and is now a standard of care in neonatology. Criteria for therapeutic hypothermia can be found at the TOBY Cooling Register Clinician's Handbook (National Perinatal Epidemiology Unit 2010)

The prognosis in this case is difficult to determine and further investigations (MRI, EEG) can help in defining outcome. Long term neurological surveillance and examination is indicated in babies who have suffered moderate or severe HIE.

34. COMMUNICATION – EXPLANATION OF BRONCHIOLITIS

Candidate's Instructions:

A 7 month old boy has attended the Emergency Department with coughing, coryza, wheezing and poor feeding. On examination he is active and alert but is wheezing a lot and has some subcostal recessions. His oxygen saturations are 89% in air but go up to 98% on nasal cannula oxygen. His older brother has similar symptoms. He was examined by the Registrar who diagnosed him with bronchiolitis and asks for the child to be admitted to the short stay ward.

You are the FY1 doctor in the paediatric team and have been asked to explain to the family that the child will need to be admitted and talk to them about his diagnosis.

With 2 minutes remaining the examiner will stop you, ask you to summarise back your findings and will ask you some direct questions.

Examiner's Instructions:

A 7 month old boy has attended ED with bronchiolitis. He is generally well but his condition is complicated by an oxygen requirement and poor oral intake that necessitates admission to the short stay ward.

The FY1 doctor in the paediatric team has been asked to explain to the family the diagnosis of bronchiolitis and the need to admit to the ward for further management.

After 6 minutes ask the candidate to conclude the discussion and ask them to name 2 investigations they would consider performing in this case.

Actor's Instructions:

Your 7 month old baby has developed coughing and wheezing over the past 2 days that has been getting worse. His 3 year old brother has had similar symptoms. You brought the baby to the hospital because he refuses to feed and you are worried that his breathing is getting worse.

Prior to this your baby has been well and you have had no health concerns about him. He was born by natural delivery at term with no problems and he is gaining weight and developing well. He is fully immunised. His brother and father are healthy. You suffer from mild asthma and you wonder whether he is developing the same.

You are very keen to go back home since it is your first day back to work tomorrow morning.

COMMUNICATION – EXPLANATION OF BRONCHIOLITIS

Task:	Achieved	Not Achieved
Introduces self		
Clarifies who they are speaking to and their relationship to child		
Sets the agenda and explains purpose of discussion		
Establishes current understanding		
Explains that symptoms are likely due to bronchiolitis		
Explains that it is viral illness causing airway inflammation		
Explains that it is not asthma although some children develop asthma later when older		
Explains that severity can vary and children can get worse before they get better		
Explains that treatment is supportive with oxygen and hydration (IV or enteral)		
Explains use of oxygen as supportive treatment		
Explains that baby needs to be admitted in view of oxygen requirement and poor feeding		
Explains that symptoms can last for up to two weeks		
Explains that once there is no further need for oxygen and feeding is better, the child can go home		
Explain there is no need for antibiotics unless evidence of underlying bacterial infection		
Give advice on bronchiolitis prevention eg through good hygiene		
Asks parent if they have any further questions		
Summarises consultation & actions from here on		
Empathetic approach		
Uses appropriate language & explains any jargon		
Offers information leaflet		
Examiner's Global Mark	/5	
Actor / Helper's Global Mark	/5	
Total Station Mark	/30	

Learning Points

Bronchiolitis is a very common condition and in most cases it is benign and resolves spontaneously. However, there is a large range of severity and the condition can become life threatening.

Additional oxygen requirement and poor hydration are the two main determinants of whether a child needs to be admitted to hospital for bronchiolitis.

Most bronchiolitis is caused by viral infection but bacterial secondary infection is a possibility. In severe cases consider investigations such as chest radiography and antibiotics if there is an obvious bacterial focus. However, most bronchiolitis treatment is supportive and investigations are not required.

35. COMMUNICATION – EXPLANATION OF NEWBORN JAUNDICE

Candidate's Instructions:

A 2 day old baby in the postnatal ward was noted to be jaundiced by the midwife. A heel prick blood test reveals that the bilirubin levels are high and that the baby will need phototherapy as a result. The child is otherwise well and exclusively breast fed. The pregnancy was unremarkable and there were no risk factors for infection.

You are the FY1 doctor in the paediatric team and have been asked to speak to the mother about neonatal jaundice and the need to commence phototherapy.

With 2 minutes remaining the examiner will stop you, ask you to summarise back your findings and will ask you some direct questions.

Examiner's Instructions:

A 2 day old breastfed baby in the postnatal ward was noted to be jaundiced and bilirubin testing has indicated that the child will need phototherapy. The baby is otherwise well.

The FY1 doctor in the paediatric team has been asked to explain to the family the diagnosis and management of neonatal jaundice.

After 6 minutes ask the candidate to conclude the discussion and ask them what further treatments they are aware of if neonatal jaundice is very severe (e.g. in the case of severe haemolysis) and does not respond to phototherapy in order to prevent kernicterus.

Actor's Instructions:

Your first baby was born yesterday and has been breastfeeding well. You had a normal pregnancy with entirely normal scans and blood tests. You delivered the baby naturally and he cried immediately after birth.

You were expecting to be discharged home but the midwife checking the baby said that he looked yellow. A doctor then did a heel prick blood test and you were told that you have to wait for the result before you go home. You heard someone say that your baby is jaundiced and remember that one of your uncles was jaundiced before he died of pancreatic cancer.

You are upset when you are told that you and the baby will need to stay on the postnatal ward for baby to receive treatment. You are happy for the treatment to be given if it is properly explained.

You are not entirely clear on what is going on and you are wondering if there is something seriously wrong with the baby. You are also keen to get home as soon as possible since it is difficult to sleep and breastfeed on the postnatal ward due to it being very noisy.

EXPLANATION – EXPLANATION OF NEWBORN JAUNDICE

Task:	Achieved	Not Achieved
Introduces self		
Clarifies who they are speaking to and relationship to child, ask for child's name		
Set the agenda and explain purpose of discussion		
Clarifies current understanding		
Explains that jaundice is caused by high bilirubin levels		
Explains that unlike in adults it is very common in newborn babies and in most cases physiological		
Explains that bilirubin is a by-product from blood breaking down. The neonatal liver cannot remove it as quickly as it happens in adults.		
Explains that breastfed babies tend to develop jaundice more but this is no reason not to breastfeed		
Explains that the baby is well but jaundice can become dangerous if bilirubin levels get too high		
Explains how phototherapy works		
Explains that baby can stay with mother and continue breastfeeding		
Explains that further blood tests will be done to exclude sinister causes of jaundice		
Explains that phototherapy will be stopped once bilirubin tests show lowering of levels		
Explains that the baby will have blood tests every 6-12 hours to determine when to stop phototherapy		
Explain that after phototherapy is stopped one last blood test will be done to ensure no rebound		
Asks parent if they have any further questions		
Summarises consultation & actions from here on		
Empathetic approach		
Uses appropriate language & explains jargon		
Offers information leaflet		
Names IVIG & exchange transfusion as available treatments for severe jaundice when asked		
Examiner's Global Mark	/5	
Actor / Helper's Global Mark	/5	
Total Station Mark	/30	

Learning Points

Neonatal jaundice is very common but always reassure the parents since phototherapy can be a traumatic intervention for them by prolonging hospital stay and interfering with breastfeeding.

Although much neonatal jaundice is completely benign remember that it can also be secondary to serious conditions such as haemolysis or sepsis. These need to be ruled out.

Control of bilirubin levels is the first priority when treating neonatal jaundice but do not underestimate the importance of maintaining contact with the mother, breastfeeding and bonding.

36. COMMUNICATION – ACUTE SURGICAL REFERRAL

Candidate's instructions:

You are an FY1 doctor in the paediatric team working in the Emergency Department.

You have just seen Ali, a 12 year old boy, who presented with a 2 day history of acute abdominal pain which started centrally and has now moved towards the right side of the abdomen. He has no diarrhoea and vomiting but does have a low grade fever. On examination he is tender in the RIF but not guarding. He has had paracetamol but is still in pain. You have inserted a cannula and sent bloods for an FBC, CRP and U&Es to the lab. Urine analysis reveals 1+ leucocytes only.

The patient's father had a ruptured appendix when he was a child and is convinced this is an evolving appendicitis and is keen for theatre ASAP. You suspect Ali has acute appendicitis and need to make referral to the surgical team on call and ask for advice about next management steps.

Examiner's instructions:

A 12 year old boy Ali has presented to the ED. He has acute right iliac fossa tenderness but no guarding but it is suggestive of appendicitis. He has had paracetamol but is still in pain. The child is currently haemodynamically stable but does have a low grade fever with no other obvious source. A cannula has been inserted and the FY1 has sent bloods to lab for FBC, CRP and U&Es. Ali's father had a ruptured appendix when he was a child and is convinced this is an evolving appendicitis and is keen for theatre ASAP.

The FY1 needs to refer the patient to the Surgical Registrar on call who is currently getting ready in theatre for an emergency operation. The FY1 doctor needs to ask the surgical team to review the patient. The FY1 also needs to ask for advice on how to manage the patient until the surgical team can see the child.

Actor's instructions:

You are Mr Yusuf, the surgical registrar on call. You are a final year registrar and have had a very busy weekend on call and you are now about to go to theatre to perform an emergency laparotomy. The theatre nurse informs you that a paediatric doctor wants to discuss a patient in the ED with you and is keen to get some advice. You are not rude or hostile but you are very pressed for time and initially wonder whether you can take the referral in an hour's time. If pressed to take the referral you want to hear the information in a short and concise manner to decide whether there is a chance of appendicitis. You are keen to check that alternative differential diagnoses have been considered.

The FY1 doctor explains she thinks the child she has just seen in the ED has appendicitis. You ask for details of the history and examination. You ask for investigation results. She reports that the blood results are outstanding but urine analysis reveals white cells only. You ask what analgesia has been given. You ask what has been explained to the child and parents.

You advise for the patient to be made nil by mouth and to be started on some maintenance IV fluids. You explain that you need to perform emergency surgery but that you agree that appendicitis is a strong possibility. You will accept the patient and ensure that your junior doctor will see the patient as soon as possible. You also ask that the parents be kept informed of the referral and that the team are coming to assess Ali further.

COMMUNICATION – ACUTE SURGICAL REFERRAL

Task	Achieved	Not achieved
Introduction and clear description of situation – 'I am the on call paediatric F1 doctor in the ED'		
Clarifies who they are speaking to (gets name and position of surgical registrar)		
Asks whether the surgical registrar is in a position to talk		
Explains urgency of referring the case now rather than delaying if asked to call back		
Explains background of child as previously fit and well		
Explains assessment - haemodynamics		
Explains assessment – abdominal examination findings		
Reinforces pain shifting from umbilicus to RIF		
States concerns about low grade fever with no other source		
Summarises interventions made and investigations sent		
Describes negative urine test to exclude UTI as an alternative		
States likely evolving appendicitis		
Informs of parental anxiety and ideas, concerns & expectations		
Clear recommendation - Requests referral to the surgical team		
Requests further management advice until team are able to see		
Confirms that patient be NBM and have maintenance fluids		
Discusses which analgesia should next be given		
Summarises the discussion		
Polite throughout conversation & thanks colleague		
Agrees to talk to parents and reassure them of active management		
Examiner's global mark	/5	
Actor's / Helper's global mark	/5	
Total station mark	/30	

Learning points:

Abdominal pain in children has a large range of differential diagnoses so careful history, examination and often periods of observation are required. Not all abdominal pains require referral to the surgeons so a clear summary in your head is required before referring on to avoid sending the child to the wrong specialty and causing potential delays.

Structure is required for referrals and SBAR – Situation, Background, Assessment and Recommendations is a well-known, useful template to follow. It is important to present things in a systematic, concise and succinct manner. This allows the person on the other end of the phone gets a clear picture of the child you have seen and this template gives you the best possible chance of doing that. Remember that it is not wrong to say 'I don't know what is going on with this child, I would like your senior opinion' as a recommendation.

The parent's ideas, concerns and expectations are important here and letting the surgeon know of their worries is important. It will not sway their decision on operating however they may mobilise a member of the team more rapidly to allay their fears and defuse any tensions for the referring team.

37. COMMUNICATION – DEMONSTRATE USE OF EPIPEN

Candidate's instructions:

You are the FY1 doctor covering the Paediatric Observation unit in ED. Reuben is a 14 year old boy who is known to the department for asthma. He presented earlier in the day following an allergic reaction to peanuts. He was at school when the reaction occurred and although he had his EpiPen with him he did not feel confident to administer it. He was given adrenaline by the paramedics. He also received antihistamine and steroids in ED. He has recovered well and but requires a period of observation before he can go home.

You saw Reuben and his father when they were admitted to the ward. You have already discussed with them about recognising mild and severe allergic reactions and which rescue medication to use for each. Reuben remains anxious and has asked if you could go over with him again when and how to use an Epipen.

Examiner's instruction:

The FY1 doctor needs to ask Reuben what his worries are. The doctor should ascertain that Reuben has concerns about having another allergic reaction and lacks confident in using his Epipen. The doctor should acknowledge Reuben's fears and try to reassure him. He should explain when Reuben needs to use an EpiPen and how to use one. Before leaving Reuben he should give him an Epipen checklist and contact details for allergy / anaphylaxis support groups.

Actor's instructions:

You are a 15 year old boy who has presented to ED with only your second episode of anaphylaxis to peanuts. The first time was when you were a toddler and you have avoided peanuts since. You are quite shaken up by this episode as you are usually very careful about what you eat. You recognised you were having an allergic reaction but didn't feel confident to make the decision to use your EpiPen. Also, you were not sure exactly how to use it.

The ward doctor spoke to you and your father when you were first admitted about how to recognise allergic reactions and when to use antihistamine and when to use your EpiPen. You can remember some of the points discussed but feel you need to go over it again for reassurance before you go home.

COMMUNICATION – DEMONSTRATE USE OF EPIPEN

Task	Achieved	Not achieved
Introduces self		
Clarifies who they are speaking to		
Establishes current understanding		
Explain managing allergies includes avoiding the allergen, antihistamine and adrenaline (EpiPen)		
Explains how to recognise an allergic reaction		
Explains difference between mild and severe symptoms		
Explains when to use antihistamine (mild symptoms ie if itching or cutaneous symptoms)		
Explains when to use Epipen (severe symptoms eg cough, breathing difficulties, feeling unwell)		
Shows how to hold pen in palm of hand and wrap hand around it in a fist with thumb tucked in		
Shows how to remove safety cap with other hand (the needle is activated when cap removed)		
Explains need to press injector tip end firmly against outer thigh until you hear 'click'. It will go through clothing that is not too thick		
Explains need to hold EpiPen in place for 10 seconds		
Explains need to remove Epipen and rub the area for another 10 seconds		
Call ambulance/ 999 after used even if feeling better (in case of biphasic reaction, may need further treatment)		
If remain unwell can use second Epipen if available (after 5 mins)		
Asks if patients has any further questions		
Summarises discussion		
Leaves patient with written allergy action plan		
Offers information leaflet		
Offers to return and explain again later if required		
Examiner's global mark /5		
Actor's / Helper's global mark /5		
Total station mark /30		

Learning points:

Signs and symptoms of allergy include:

Mild	Severe (in addition to mild symptoms)
Sneezing, runny or blocked nose,	Feeling lightheaded or faint
Red, itchy, watery eyes,	Swelling of mouth, throat or tongue may cause breathing or swallowing difficulties
Red, itchy rash	Wheezing or coughing
Swollen eyelids or lips	Abdominal pain, nausea and vomiting
Worsening of eczema	Collapse and unconsciousness

Anaphylaxis is an emergency and can be a frightening experience for children. It is important that parents and children realise that EpiPens can be life-saving treatment. Key points to include when discussing EpiPens:

Those at risk of anaphylaxis or their parents should always carry two EpiPens and antihistamine with them at all times. They should ensure that EpiPens are not expired and should be replaced as needed. If they are expired the advice is to still use them in an emergency but be aware it may not be effective. The pen should be stored at room temperature. Used pens must be replaced as soon as possible.

Lie child down with feet elevated if they tolerate it. If child has symptoms of wheeze and have their reliever inhaler they can take that also.

Parents and child should be aware that they will need to be monitored in hospital for several hours afterwards after being treated for anaphylaxis. If it is their first episode some children may be admitted overnight.

38. COMMUNICATION – DEMONSTRATE USE OF INHALER AND SPACER

Candidate's instructions

You are an FY1 doctor on the General Paediatric ward. Iris, a 2 year old girl, was admitted two days ago with acute viral wheeze requiring nebulised salbutamol. Iris is being discharged home today. You have been asked by your team to explain and demonstrate how to use a metered dose inhaler (MDI) with a mask and spacer to the parent who is anxious about going home.

Iris is not by the bedside. You can use a nearby doll or teddy bear to demonstrate inhaler + spacer + mask technique to the parent.

Examiner's instruction

The candidate will be expected to demonstrate to a parent how to use an inhaler with a mask and spacer and how to clean the spacer and mask. They should introduce themselves and confirm who they are speaking to. They should elicit parent's prior knowledge. They should acknowledge the parents anxiety.

They should use one of Iris's teddy bears / dolls to demonstrate to how to use an MDI with an age appropriate spacer and mask. They should explain how to clean the spacer and mask. They should summarise their discussion. They should offer the parent written information. They should ask if parent has any questions and also offer parent opportunity to have a further discussion before discharge.

Actor's instruction:

You are the parent of Iris who was admitted for the first time two days ago with viral wheeze following a cold. She has had similar episodes of wheeze on her chest before but has not previously been so severe. You are anxious about stopping the nebulisers and going home with just the inhalers and spacers.

The FY1 doctor has come to see you while Iris is spending time with the play specialist. You have seen them before on the ward round these last couple of days. You tell the doctor that you've seen the inhaler and spacer before at home but that your partner usually gives it to Iris if she needs it.

COMMUNICATION – DEMONSTRATE USE OF INHALER AND SPACER

Task	Achieved	Not achieved
Introduces self with name and position		
Clarifies who they are speaking to		
Establishes previous knowledge of inhaler/spacer usage		
Acknowledges parent's concerns		
Explains when inhaler/spacer should be used		
Explains that inhaler with spacer is a very effective way of delivering salbutamol in children		
Demonstrates need to shake inhaler for 5 seconds (this helps mix medicine with propellant) and then place into spacer		
Shows how to position / hold child (cuddles child on your lap facing away from them)		
Demonstrates how to put mask on face to get good seal and avoid eye area		
Shows how to press once on canister to release one dose/puff of medication		
Shows ned to allow child to breathe normally for 10 seconds with mask in place		
Removes mask and waits approximately one minute before repeating dose if required		
Explains need to clean monthly or if visibly dirty		
Shows how to clean with lukewarm water and mild soap		
Explains need to allow to drip dry		
Summarises discussion		
Offers written information (wheeze management plan)		
Suggests reputable websites for further information e.g. Asthma UK		
Asks if mother has any other questions now		
Offers to come back and discuss again later if parent has more questions		
Examiner's global mark		
Actor's / Helper's global mark		
Total station mark		

Learning points:

The inhaler and spacer (+ mask) is a very effective technique at delivering medicine. The medicine gets straight into the lungs where it is needed and quickly too. In addition there are less side effects as not much medicine is absorbed to the rest of body. MDIs with a spacer are easier to use as the spacer collects the medicine inside them, so the parent does not have to worry about pressing the inhaler and child having to breathe in at exactly the same time.

Many children with asthma are prescribed two different types of asthma inhaler: a daily preventer inhaler to help protect their airways and reduce the chance of triggers causing asthma symptoms and a reliever inhaler for immediate relief of symptoms. As the child gets bigger inhalers and spacers might need to change. The child should see the asthma nurse or GP every 6 months for an asthma review.

When teaching a parent/patient a new technique it is important to initially demonstrate that technique yourself. Allow enough time for the parent (patient) to practice with you helping them and then ask them to demonstrate to you the technique or repeat the instructions back to you.

39. COMMUNICATION – EXPLAIN MANAGEMENT OF ECZEMA TO A PARENT

Candidate's Instructions

You are a FY1 doctor sitting in the Paediatric Outpatient Clinic. The next patient is Magda, a 3 year old girl, has come with her mother to clinic. Magda has had eczema for the last year. Her mother has tried a number of organic creams and soaps from the health food shop but none of these have helped and recently Magda's skin has worsened. Magda's eczema is now also beginning to affect her sleep and she is very irritable and uncomfortable during the day. Her mother is at her wit's end and has come to see you to see what treatments are available to help Magda.

The consultant feels Magda needs medical treatment and hands Magda's mother, Louisa, a prescription. While the consultant takes an important phone call in another room she asks if you would kindly talk through the treatments with Magda's mother.

Examiner's instructions

A mother has bought her 3 year old daughter Magda to the Paediatric Outpatient Clinic. Magda has eczema and her mother has not yet tried any medications to help control her symptoms instead seeking advice from health food shops and trying a number of natural organic soaps and creams. Magda's eczema has worsened and now her mother feels she needs to try prescription creams. The FY1 doctor needs to explain what the skin condition eczema is. The FY1 needs to explain how to use emollients and how to use topical steroids and also mention rare side effects of topical steroids. The FY1 should direct the mother to helpful websites and also give written information about the treatment of eczema including how to fingertip units of steroid.

Actor's instructions

You are Louisa. Magda is your only child. Magda has had eczema for the last year. You initially wanted to avoid any unnecessary medications and so you sought help from your local health food shop and have tried a number of organic and natural soaps and creams. These did not appear to help and some actually made Magda's eczema worse. Magda has recently been very irritable at night, scratching her skin a lot causing it to bleed at times. She is finding it difficult to sleep through the night and this is also affecting her daytime wellbeing. You spoke with your husband and after a long discussion have finally come to seek help from the doctor. You have some reservations but realise that you now need to get Magda's eczema under control.

COMMUNICATION – EXPLAIN MANAGEMENT OF ECZEMA TO A PARENT

Task	Achieved	Not achieved
Introduces self		
Clarifies whom they are speaking to and relationship to child		
Clarifies current knowledge/understanding		
Explains what eczema is (inflammation of the skin) leading to skin that is hot, red, itchy and dry.		
Explains no cure and that treatment involves controlling and easing symptoms		
Explains eczema can be triggered by change in weather, stress, illnesses and food allergies or sensitivities to pollen, house dust mite or pet dander.		
Treatments include avoiding triggers, emollients (moisturisers) and topical corticosteroids.		
Keeping nails short and wearing soft clothes made from cotton can help symptoms.		
Parents should avoid soaps that irritate skin (perfumes and colourants can exacerbate eczema). Instead can use soap substitutes.		
Emollients are lotions, creams or ointments made of a mixture of oil and water. They create a protective barrier on the top layer of skin and help reduce water loss.		
Should apply emollients at least 2-4 times a day		
Wash hands prior to applying emollients. If no pump dispenser available, use spoon		
Apply large amount to skin and smooth down (not rub in) in direction of hair.		
Topical corticosteroids treat inflammation of the skin		
Leave at least 10 minutes gap between emollient and steroid		
Apply steroids only to inflamed areas of skin (as often as instructed, usually once a day)		
One adult fingertip unit enough to cover twice size of adult hands (or use fingertip unit chart)		
Rare topical steroid side effects (more likely if using strong steroid for many months, using in sensitive areas such as face and groin, and using		

large amounts): thinning of skin, changes in skin colour (although this is also associated with inflammation), increased hair growth.		
Draws attention to useful websites (NHS choices, Patient UK) and offers written information including fingertip unit guide		
Asks if further questions and summarises		
Examiner's global mark	/5	
Actor's / Helper's global mark	/5	
Total station mark	/30	

Learning points

If you are presented with a young baby with severe eczema consideration needs to be given to possible cow's milk protein allergy. In addition, if a baby presents with eczema for the first time around weaning then a feeding history is imperative to help pinpoint any food triggers for the eczema. If the subsequent management includes food exclusion then the input of a paediatric dietician should be sought.

Eczematous skin is prone to infection. Features of infected skin include weeping blisters, pustules, crusting, not responding to usual treatment, and rapidly worsening eczema. If the infected area is small, a topical antibiotic may be used. More widespread infection will need treatment with oral antibiotics.

If treatment with emollients and topical corticosteroids is not sufficient to control symptoms, children can be referred on for more specialist treatment such as wet bandages, phototherapy, steroid sparing agents (topical calcineurin inhibitors), very strong corticosteroids, and immunosuppressant therapy.

40. COMMUNICATION – EXPLAIN DIAGNOSIS OF TRISOMY 21 TO A PARENT

Candidate's instructions:

You are an FY1 doctor working on the postnatal ward with the Paediatric team. You are carrying out routine newborn baby checks when the senior midwife on the ward approaches you and asks if you would kindly speak to a mother who was yesterday informed her new baby son Simon is likely to have Down's Syndrome. She is anxious and has some questions she would like to ask.

Examiner's instructions:

A mother on the postnatal ward was told yesterday that her newborn son shows signs of Down's Syndrome. She is awaiting the results of a genetic test to confirm the diagnosis. She is very worried and has lots of questions she would like answered. The FY1 should tell the mother the immediate concerns (to rule out congenital cardiac anomaly, check for hypothyroidism, to establish feeding). The FY1 should outline long term problems. The FY1 should explain about referral to community paediatrics and the MDT. The FY1 should offer to chase results, get seniors to come back to talk to mother and offer written information. The FY1 should also direct the mother to Down Syndrome support groups.

Actor's instructions:

You are a 37 year old woman on the postnatal ward and your baby boy Simon was born yesterday morning by normal vaginal delivery. He is your first child born at term. You had an uneventful pregnancy and as far as you know, both of your antenatal scans were normal. You did not have any additional tests during pregnancy to assess for Down's as you felt the risk was low despite your age. You have no past medical history and only take the vitamin supplements you were given during pregnancy. You are a non-smoker and a very occasional drinker but have not had any during pregnancy. Your husband is very supportive and has been very excited about the birth.

After Simon was born the midwife had some concerns about his appearance and asked the paediatrician to come and speak to you. The paediatrician agreed that Simon showed signs of Down Syndrome and asked permission to do a genetic test to confirm the diagnosis of which the results are now awaited.

You are feeling very guilty for not having more tests during pregnancy and are not sure how you and your husband will cope with this unexpected news. You are too scared to look on the internet to find out more about the condition but have heard of Down Syndrome and think it means Simon will be quite disabled. You've let your midwife know of your concerns and she has asked another paediatric doctor to come and speak to you.

You would like to know how Simon will be affected both now and in the long term. You would like to know what help there will be for Simon and most importantly when the results would be back.

COMMUNICATION – EXPLAIN DIAGNOSIS OF TRISOMY 21 TO A PARENT

Task	Achieved	Not achieved
Introduces self with name and position		
Clarifies who they are speaking to & how they can help		
Allows mother time and space to talk when tearful		
Empathises with mother as to why she is feeling anxious		
Establishes current understanding of Trisomy 21		
Explains that antenatal scan may not always show signs of Down's		
Explains concisely Down Syndrome is – genetic condition with extra chromosome		
Explains what immediate management goals are while inpatient – establish feeding, blood tests (TSH) to detect hypothyroidism, echocardiogram to rule out congenital anomalies.		
Explains referral to community paediatrics will occur		
Explains involvement of a MDT (SALT, Physio, OT, dietician)		
Explains some potential long term problems – developmental delay, learning difficulties, hearing and visual problems		
Explains some people with Down Syndrome go to mainstream school, have employment, live independently.		
Explains there will be planned regular reviews		
Offers to chase up genetic test result		
Offers seniors to return to discuss with parents		
Offers written information		
Directs mother to patient support group		
Asks if mother has any other questions now		
Summarises discussion		
Offers to come back and discuss again later if parent has more questions		
Examiner's global mark	/5	
Actor's / Helper's global mark	/5	
Total station mark	/30	

Learning points:

Down syndrome is not preventable but can be screened for antenatally. The screening involves blood tests and measurements from ultrasound to work out the chance of a baby being born with Down's Syndrome. The combined test is offered in early pregnancy (10-14 weeks) and the quad test is offered later (14-20 weeks). Diagnostic tests include CVS and Amniocentesis.

It is important to be honest when giving parents a diagnosis. If you can't answer their questions say you will find out and get back to them or that you will get a senior to talk to them. Try not to overload them with too much information.

When giving a new diagnosis to a patient / parents there are a number of key points to always follow: arrange for further discussion another time, give written information if available and direct them to patient support groups.

CLINICAL SKILLS

41. CLINICAL SKILLS - INTERPRET A BLOOD GAS

Candidate's instructions

Tabitha is a 12 year old girl brought by ambulance to hospital after she was found unconscious in her room. She had had a two day history of feeling unwell with a 'tummy bug' and had stayed off school that day. She was previously fit and well.

IV access is gained and venous blood samples taken including a blood gas.

```
BLOOD GAS ANALYSER

JONES, Tabitha
Hospital number: 765432
DOB 02/02/2004

Details:
Sample: venous
Temp: 37.0 C
FiO2: 21%

pH          7.05              (7.35 - 7.45)
PCO₂        2.5     kPa       (4.5 - 6.1)
PO₂         5.6     kPa       (11 - 13)
Na⁺         131     mmol/L    (135 - 145)
K⁺          5.2     mmol/L    (3.5 - 5.0)
Cl⁻         106     mmol/L    (99 - 107)
Ca²⁺        1.32    mmol/L    (1.1 - 1.35)
Glu         43      mmol/L    (4 - 7)
Lac         2.5     mmol/L    (0.5 - 2)
Hb          185     g/L       (120 - 170)
saO₂        56      %
HCO₃⁻       9.5     mmol/L    (22 - 26)
BE          -22
```

Please interpret her venous blood gas results and present your findings, explaining your rationale:

Examiner's instructions

Tabitha is a 12 year old girl brought by ambulance to hospital after she was found unconscious in her room. She had had a two day history of feeling unwell with a 'tummy bug' and had stayed off school that day. She was previously fit and well.

The candidate is presented with the results of a venous blood gas including normal values for arterial samples. Please allow the candidate TWO minutes to study the blood gas and then prompt as follows:

'Would you like to present your findings to me please?'
'Please suggest the most likely diagnosis for Tabitha's presentation'
'Can you think of any differential diagnoses for comatose presentation with this type of acid base disturbance?'
'Why will Tabitha's potassium will need careful monitoring over the next 24 hours?'
'What is the greatest risk to Tabitha if her fluid balance is not well controlled?'

CLINICAL SKILLS - INTERPRET A BLOOD GAS

Task	Achieved	Not achieved
Introduces presentation with patient demographics		
Identifies severe acidosis		
Identifies acidosis is metabolic in nature		
Identifies extremely low bicarbonate and large base deficit		
Identifies low pCO2		
Mentions this low pCO2 is partial respiratory compensation		
Comments on pO2 / Sa O2 – low as it is a venous sample		
Recognises high glucose		
Identifies slightly raised lactate – unlikely to be significantly contributing to the acidosis		
Recognises high anion gap acidosis (AG = 21)		
Recognises hyponatraemia		
Recognises hyperkalaemia		
Identifies high haemoglobin as likely secondary to intravascular dehydration		
Concise and logical presentation		
Summarises key positive findings in one – two sentences		
Discusses differential diagnosis for high anion gap acidosis (lactic, keto-acidosis, toxins e.g. salicylate, paracetamol)		
Single most likely diagnosis: diabetic ketoacidosis (new presentation type 1 diabetes mellitus) (2 marks)		
Potassium will fall as insulin is commenced		
Fluid balance needs to be well controlled due to high risk of cerebral oedema		
Examiner's mark	/5	
Total station mark	/25	

Learning points

It is important to use a structured approach to interpreting and presenting a blood gas:

Is the pH acidotic or alkalotic?

Check the pCO2: It is high in a respiratory acidosis or compensated metabolic alkalosis. It is low in a respiratory alkalosis or compensated metabolic acidosis.

Check the HCO3- and base excess to see if it confirms a metabolic component to the blood gas result. There will be a large negative base excess in a metabolic acidosis, or a positive excess in a metabolic alkalosis. Alternatively, it may show evidence of compensatory mechanisms, to respiratory acidosis or alkalosis.

Following this you can use the other parameters on the blood gas (lactate, electrolytes, haemoglobin, glucose) to gather a lot of useful information regarding the cause of the disturbance and put the acid base disturbance you have identified in context.

Calculation of the anion gap is useful in emergency situations where there is a severe metabolic acidosis and unclear cause – make sure you know how to calculate it and the causes of high and normal anion gap. The normal range for the anion gap is 8 – 16 mmol/l. Remember that in this situation of DKA the anion gap will be underestimated as the true sodium is likely higher (see below).

Anion gap = (sodium + potassium) – (bicarbonate + chloride)

Sodium is particularly important to monitor in the first 24 hours of DKA management. Severe hyperglycaemia causes osmotic shift of water from the intracellular space into the extracellular space. This leads to a relative dilutional hyponatraemia, so 'true' body sodium will be higher that the lab values suggest. Subsequently, as glucose is driven back into cells with insulin, the diffusion gradient is reversed, allowing water back into the intracellular space. This can potentially cause cerebral oedema with devastating consequences. Therefore, sodium levels are checked frequently during initial management to ensure rehydration is not too rapid. A correction equation comprising the lab sodium and blood glucose can ascertain the 'true' sodium.

Corrected sodium = measured Na^+ + 0.4 ([glucose] – 5.5)

42. CLINICAL SKILLS - INTERPRET A CHEST X-RAY

Candidate's instructions

Jason is a 2 week old baby who has attended ED with a three day history of poor feeding, coryza and increasing respiratory distress. On examination there are fine crackles and wheeze throughout with reduced air entry in the right upper zone.

Please assess his Chest X-ray and present your findings.

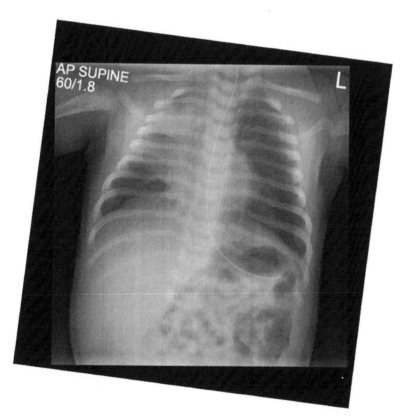

Examiner's instructions

Jason is a 2 week old baby who has attended ED with a three day history of poor feeding, coryza and increasing respiratory distress. On examination there are fine crackles and wheeze throughout with reduced air entry in the right upper zone.

The candidate is asked to look at the X-ray and present their findings. Please give the candidate TWO minutes to assess the image then prompt their assessment:

'Would you like to present your findings?'

After the candidate's presentation of the image, please prompt as follows:

'Given the history and Chest X-ray findings, what would your top two differential diagnoses be?'

'What other investigations would you like to perform?'

'What normal structure is often seen in Chest X-rays of babies as a smooth mass in the superior mediastinum?'

CLINICAL SKILLS - INTERPRET A CHEST X-RAY

Task	Achieved	Not achieved
Logical, concise presentation		
Confirms patient's name		
Confirms patient's date of birth		
Confirms patient's hospital number		
Comments on limitations of AP and supine film		
Comments on inspiration (adequate)		
Comments on rotation (adequate, possibly a little to left)		
Comments on exposure (adequate)		
Comments on artefact: NG tube sited correctly within the stomach bubble		
Comments on heart size: cannot assess fully with AP film but looks <50% of cardiothoracic ratio		
Comments on bones and soft tissue (normal)		
Comments on lung parenchyma (generalised prominence of bronchovascular markings, especially in the perihilar region – consistent with inflammatory process)		
Comments on costophrenic angles (normal)		
Comments on focal lung abnormality – consolidation +/- collapse of right middle and upper lobes (loss of definition at apex and right heart border, slight loss of lung volume, potential mediastinal shift)		
Comments on visible bowel gas pattern		
Comments on important negatives (nil pleural effusion, no focal change on left)		
Summarises important positive findings in 1-2 sentences		
Suggests appropriate differential diagnosis: bronchiolitis with right middle & upper lobe collapse / consolidation, secondary bacterial LRTI affecting right mid/upper lobe		
Other investigations: inflammatory markers, respiratory viral screen, blood culture, sputum culture if able, capillary blood gas		
Normal mass in mediastinum: thymus		
Examiner's mark	/5	
Global mark	/25	

Learning points

Regardless of the standout abnormality on any Chest X-ray, you need a logical system for interpreting a film which encompasses all the points above (bones, soft tissues, NG tube placement etc). Otherwise you will miss important but subtle findings.

Bronchiolitis is caused by viral pathogens but can have dramatic Chest X-ray changes, often including consolidation or collapse of the right upper lobe.

It is very difficult to distinguish on paediatric Chest X-rays between bacterial and viral changes, especially as viral respiratory tract infections can lead to secondary bacterial pneumonias. Correlation with clinical findings and laboratory investigations is essential.

43. CLINICAL SKILLS - VENEPUNCTURE IN AN OLDER CHILD

Candidate's instructions

You are an FY1 doctor in Paediatric ED. You have clerked Ryan, a 15 year old presenting with a petechial rash and atraumatic bruising who is otherwise well. After discussing with the registrar, a plan is made to do some blood tests to check platelet count and clotting profile. Ryan's mother has left the department for 10 minutes to get a coffee.

Please explain the procedure to Ryan, gain verbal consent and perform venepuncture using the equipment provided.

Examiner's instructions

Ryan is a 15 year old with atraumatic bruising and petechial rash who needs a blood test in ED. His mother has left for a coffee so the FY1 gains verbal consent from Ryan in her absence and performs the procedure.

After 6 minutes, ask the candidate to finish the procedure and ask:

What resources for distraction therapy might be useful in a younger child?

Actor's instructions:

You are Ryan, a 15 year old boy with some bruising and a purple pinprick rash that have come out of nowhere after a cold last week. You are nervous about being in ED as it's noisy with lots of crying children and you've never had to come to hospital before. However, you feel like you should act grown up to prove to everyone that you don't really need to be in the children's area.

You think you might have had a blood test when you were a baby but you can't remember it. Last year when you had a vaccination at school you remember your arm hurt for days afterwards (though that might have been because your friends kept punching it). If the doctor explains to you why the blood test is needed you will agree to have it done and will be fine without your mum present. If offered, you would like to try the cold spray as long as you can test what it feels like first.

CLINICAL SKILLS - VENEPUNCTURE IN OLDER CHILD

Task:	Achieved	Not Achieved
Introduces self		
Confirms identity of patient		
Asks whether he would like to wait for his mother		
Establishes prior knowledge of procedure		
Explains why a blood test needed		
Explains the process step by step		
Is truthful regarding pain involved in procedure		
Offers topical anaesthesia (cream / cold spray)		
Asks if child has any other concerns or questions		
Obtains verbal confirmation of consent		
Assembles equipment (tourniquet, butterfly needle, vacutainer, plaster, 70% alcohol wipe, cold spray, blood bottles)		
Appropriate decontamination of hands and puts on gloves		
Applies tourniquet		
Identifies suitable vein		
Secure hold of limb and stretch of skin		
Cleans skin and does not recontaminate		
Successfully aspirates blood via vacutainer		
Disposes of needle into sharps bin safely		
Appropriate post procedure care (apply pressure for 30 seconds, then apply plaster, ensures child is comfortable)		
Distraction therapy: books, smartphones, play therapist, bubbles, noisy toys		
Examiner's Global Mark	/5	
Actor / Helper's Global Mark	/5	
Total Station Mark	/30	

Learning points:

Teenagers often look more mature than they are and hide their anxiety well – do not assume they have had a blood test before. Always offer to wait for their parent and to use cold spray (with topical anaesthetic cream if very anxious).

Be truthful – don't say it won't hurt when you know it will! Do try to help them contextualise and rationalise this (you will only feel a sharp scratch for a short time / we can count down from 10 if you like / it won't hurt as much as when you last stubbed your toe)

Distraction therapy is often used alongside topical analgesia in the younger age group (and often more effective!) – this can include smartphone games, noisy toys, bubbles, picture books and singing songs. Play therapists and nursing staff are invaluable in this role.

44. CLINICAL SKILLS - ADMINISTER INTRAMUSCULAR INJECTION

Candidate's instructions

You are the FY1 doctor on the Special Care Baby Unit. Benjy, an ex 32 week premature baby is now 8 weeks old and due his first set of routine immunisations.

Please obtain verbal consent from his mother and perform the task using the equipment provided.

Examiner's instructions

Benjy, an ex 32 week premature baby on the Special Care Baby Unit is now 8 weeks old and due his first set of routine immunisations.

The FY1 doctor on the team has been asked to obtain verbal consent from his mother and then perform the task using the equipment provided.

During the practical component, ask regarding landmarks in infants for intramuscular injections.

If the following has not been mentioned prior, at 6 minutes, ask the candidate to complete the procedure and ask:
1.   Can you think of any complications of intramuscular injections you would mention to the parents?
2.   What side effects of vaccinations would you warn the parents to expect?

Actor's instructions

You are the mother of Benjy, an ex premature baby (32 weeks gestation) who is still in the Special Care Baby Unit but is now 8 weeks old. He is due his routine 8 week immunisations today.

You have no particular objections to your baby having immunisations but wonder if there are any oral formulations of the vaccines that he could have instead because he's had to endure so many needles so far. If the doctor mentions that he may be unwell with a fever after the vaccinations, you should ask whether that means he will need antibiotics as he has received three courses of intravenous antibiotics over the past 8 weeks for similar reasons.

You would like to know if there are any other likely complications as a result of these injections.

CLINICAL SKILLS - ADMINISTER INTRAMUSCULAR INJECTION

Task:	Achieved	Not Achieved
Introduces self		
Clarifies who they are speaking to and relationship to child		
Establishes current understanding of procedure		
Explains intramuscular injections provide a depot for the drug / vaccine to dissipate through the body over a longer time		
Lists complications: Common - tenderness at local site. Rare - bleeding, infection, inadvertent iv administration		
Explains fever and malaise common after immunisations – manage with paracetamol, needs clinical review or antibiotics if other additional symptoms		
Asks if parent has any other concerns or questions		
Obtains verbal consent		
Assembles equipment (appropriate gauge needle, syringe, plaster, 70% alcohol wipe)		
Confirms name and DOB of baby on ID band and with mother		
Confirms allergy status		
Checks drug dose and expiry date with colleague		
Appropriate decontamination of hands and puts on gloves		
Does not recontaminate		
Appropriate site (middle third of thigh preferred, can also use deltoid muscle)		
Takes secure hold of child's limb		
Inserts needle at 90 degree angle to skin		
Aspirates prior to injecting		
Discards needle into sharps bin safely		
Appropriate post procedure care (check for bleeding, apply plaster, ensures child is comfortable)		
Examiner's Global Mark	/5	
Actor / Helper's Global Mark	/5	
Total Station Mark	/30	

Learning points

The middle third of the thigh is the best place for intramuscular injections in babies as this is the location of largest muscle mass. The deltoid muscle can also be used. Each injection should be at a different site.

Remember to anticipate a struggle and secure the limb well before you start to minimize risk of needlestick injury to yourself and distress to the child.

If administering vaccinations in a hospital setting, details of the immunisation (brand, lot, expiry, site and date) should be recorded in the drug chart, the hospital notes and the red book.

45. CLINICAL SKILLS - ACUTE ASTHMA

Candidate's Instructions:

An 8 year old boy who is a known asthmatic has presented to the Emergency Department with shortness of breath.

You are the FY1 doctor in the Paediatric team and have been asked to complete the initial assessment and suggest appropriate treatment as necessary.

Examiner's Instructions:

An 8 year old boy has been brought to the emergency department with a 1 day history of worsening shortness of breath.

The FY1 Paediatric doctor has been asked to complete the initial assessment of the patient, which they should do in an A to E approach, suggesting appropriate treatment as they go along.

On arrival the child is alert but finding it difficult to complete sentences.

Initial observations: Saturations 91% in air, RR-35, HR-130, T-36.5. He has tracheal tug with intercostal recessions and is sitting leaning forward. On auscultation of the chest he has scattered wheeze. Please offer observations as requested by candidate.

He does not respond to the first nebuliser and therefore back-to-back nebulisers should be given as well as oral prednisolone.
On re-assessment after back-to-back nebulisers he has the following observations: Sats-89% in air (or 97% in 8L/min high flow O_2), RR-32, HR-135. He still has tracheal tug with intercostal recessions. On auscultation of the chest he is still wheezy throughout.

At this stage it would be appropriate for the candidate to consider IV therapy, as the child is not responding well and at risk of deterioration. They should also call for senior support as this child has acute severe asthma.

He is accompanied by his mother who is upset and asks whether her child is going to be ok. The candidate should answer her question and explain their management.

After 6 minutes please stop the candidate and ask them to summarise their assessment and management plan.

Actor's Instructions:

You have brought your 8-year-old boy to the emergency department who has a 1 day history of worsening shortness of breath. He started with coryzal symptoms 3 days ago and has had a non-productive cough for the past 2 days that is worse at night. He hasn't had any fevers but has been more lethargic today and not eaten or drunk much.

He was diagnosed with asthma at 6 years of age after recurrent episodes of wheeze in the winter. He has been admitted to hospital 3 times in the past year, requiring intravenous therapy on two occasions but never being admitted to PICU.

His consultant escalated his asthma treatment 2 months ago, however he is not very compliant with his medication. Cold weather triggers his asthma as well as animal fur. He has eczema and both you and your other son suffer with asthma too. He has no known drug allergies but is allergic to nuts and fish. Otherwise he has no other medical history.

On arrival to the ED he is breathless and finding it difficult to complete sentences. You are scared and want to make sure he is going to be ok. After the first nebuliser you can see he is still working hard with his breathing and is breathless. The back-to-back nebulisers help a little but he says his chest still feels tight.

After the intravenous therapy his chest starts to feel a bit better and he is able to talk more easily.

Your feel very anxious as he has been unwell lots of times before, but it helps when the doctor reassures you.

CLINICAL SKILLS STATION OSCE - Acute Asthma

Task:	Achieved	Not Achieved
Introduces self to patient/parent		
Checks correct patient name and DOB (with patient or parent)		
Assesses airway patency		
Gives high flow oxygen via facemask		
Attaches pulse oximeter (aim 94-98%)		
Assesses Respiratory rate		
Assesses effort of breathing		
Auscultates chest		
Assesses Heart rate		
Assesses CRT, BP, Temp		
Assesses level of consciousness (AVPU scale)		
Gives beta-2-agonists and ipratropium bromide via nebuliser (NB: through oxygen)		
Gives oral prednisolone		
Re-assesses patient after initial treatment		
States would give back to back nebulisers		
Re-assesses patient after back to back nebulisers		
States would call for senior help/peri-arrest call as patient not clinically improving		
States would give IV therapy (salbutamol, magnesium sulphate or aminophylline) as patient not responded to nebulisers		
Reassures patient and parent, explaining management		
Systematic approach to assessing and managing a child with acute severe asthma		
Examiner's Global Mark	/5	
Actor / Helper's Global Mark	/5	
Total Station Mark	/30	

Learning Points

Have a clear ABCDE approach to any child with breathing difficulties. Ensure you take time to elicit all the essential parameters especially respiratory rate, and saturations (Resuscitation Council UK 2016)

Ensure you call for senior help at any early stage as asthmatic children can deteriorate quickly.

Do not forget to regularly re-assess and check response to treatment before escalating management.

Further guidance on how to manage acute asthma is available from the British Thoracic Society (British Thoracic Society 2016).

46. CLINICAL SKILLS - CARDIAC ARREST

Candidate's Instructions:

A parent on the ward has rushed out of their cubicle shouting that their child "is not waking up".

You are the Paediatric FY1 covering the ward and have been fast-bleeped by the nurse to urgently assess this child and start treatment.

Examiner's Instructions:

A 4 year old boy being treated for pneumonia on the children's ward has become unresponsive. He was admitted that day and is being treated with intravenous antibiotics. He has been gradually deteriorating and from his observation chart it would appear that the patient is septic.

The FY1 doctor has been fast-bleeped to urgently assess him as the rest of the team is attending a neonatal emergency. They should initially open the child's airway, assess for signs of life and responsiveness, before following the cardiac arrest algorithm. The candidate should ask for a cardiac arrest call (2222, Paediatric Cardiac Arrest) to be made.

The initial rhythm (once the pads are placed) is PEA and so adrenaline should be given followed by chest compressions being quickly re-commenced. At next assessment the rhythm remains unchanged and so reversible causes must be considered. After a further 2 minute cycle the rhythm is VF, at this stage the candidate must prepare for and then give an asynchronous DC shock. This successfully converts the patient back into sinus rhythm and the candidate should then discontinue CPR and state they would give post cardiac arrest treatment, including referral and transfer to PICU.

The mother is understandably distraught and initially angry that the doctors have not seen her son sooner. Ask the candidate how best they would deal with that situation?

After 6 minutes please stop the candidate and ask them to summarise their initial treatment and further management.

Actor's Instructions:

Your 4 year old son has been admitted to the children's ward today with pneumonia after being unwell for the past 2 days with high fevers, cough and difficulty in breathing. He is being treated with intravenous antibiotics and facemask oxygen, which the nurses seem to keep turning up. He has only really had 2 cups of water in the past 2 days and he keeps vomiting, so the nurses are waiting for the doctor to come and prescribe some fluids.

You have been really worried about him for the past hour as he is becoming more drowsy. You just went out of the room for 1 minute and have come back and now he is not responding to you.

He was born at 29 weeks gestation, and has chronic lung disease, requiring home oxygen for the first year of life. He has been admitted to PICU at 9 months of age with bronchiolitis but not again since then. He has no history of cardiac defects or other medical problems and has only been admitted to hospital once in the past year for a chest infection. He has some mild motor developmental delay. He is attending nursery and is up to date with his immunisations.

CLINICAL SKILLS - CARDIAC ARREST

Task:	Achieved	Not Achieved
Introduces self		
Assesses response by gently shaking and calling patient's name		
Manually opens airway (Head tilt, chin lift)		
Checks if patient is breathing for 10 seconds		
Gives 5 rescue breaths using bag-valve mask		
Assesses for signs of life		
Palpates central pulse for 10 seconds		
Recognises cardiac arrest and commences CPR at rate of 100-120 per minute		
Asks team member to put out paediatric cardiac arrest call		
Asks team member (once available) to manage airway then instigates compression:ventilation ratio of 15:2		
Asks team member to attach defibrillation pads and then stops CPR to assess rhythm		
Correctly gives adrenaline (0.1ml/kg of 1:10,000) as Pulseless Electrical Activity (PEA) identified		
Continues CPR for 2 minute cycle and then re-assesses rhythm		
Recommences CPR as still PEA		
Considers reversible causes (4Hs and 4Ts)		
Re-assesses rhythm after 2 minute cycle		
Recognises 'shockable rhythm' and appropriately deliver shock. Recommences CPR immediately		
Recognises return of spontaneous circulation and states will commence 'post cardiac arrest treatment'		
Allocates staff member to support parents		
Systematic approach to cardiac arrest in the child		
Examiner's Global Mark	/5	
Actor / Helper's Global Mark	/5	
Total Station Mark	/30	

Learning Points

'Non-shockable rhythms' (asystole or PEA) are a more common finding in children in cardiac arrest compared with 'shockable rhythms' (VF or pulseless VT). It is important you know how to manage the sequence of events for both pathways and also when to give cardiac drugs.

Drug	Dose	Route	Given
Adrenaline	10micrograms/kg 0.1ml/kg	IV/IO	Immediately with PEA/Asystole then every 4 minutes After 3rd shock if VF/pulseless VT, then after every alternate shock
Amiodarone	5mg/kg	IV/IO	After 3rd and 5th DC shock only
Lidocaine (alternative to amiodarone if unavailable)	1mg/kg	IV/IO	After 3rd and 5th DC shock only
Magnesium	25-50mg/kg	IV/IO	Polymorphic VT (torsades de pointes)

Be able to list the reversible causes for cardiac arrest (4Hs and 4Ts) but remember the most common causes in children are hypoxia and hypovolaemia.

'4Hs'	'4Ts'
Hypoxia	Thromboembolism (pulmonary or coronary)
Hypovolaemia	Tension pneumothorax
Hyper/hypokalaemia, and other Metabolic disturbances	Tamponade (cardiac)
Hypothermia	Toxic/therapeutic disturbance

It is very uncommon for children to have a cardiac arrest, but when it does happen it can be very upsetting for all the team involved. Ensure you make the time for a debrief session and seek the support you need. Further information is available from the Resuscitation Council UK website (Resuscitation Council UK 2015)

47. CLINICAL SKILLS - GROWTH CHARTS

Candidate's Instructions:

You are the FY1 in Paediatrics and have been asked to plot the growth parameters of a 13 month-old boy that has been referred into hospital by the nurse practitioner with concerns about poor weight gain.

Please advise which measurements you would like and how to measure them followed by plotting them on the appropriate growth chart.

You will be given his birth parameters for comparison.

Examiner's Instructions

A 13 month old boy has been brought in by his mum for growth assessment as the nurse practitioner is concerned about poor weight gain.

The candidate has been asked to explain to mum which growth parameters they would like to take and how these will be measured.

They should request the following:
1.   Weight (specifying without clothes or nappy)
2.   Length (specifying without nappy and using measuring board/mat)
3.   Head circumference (specifying they should take three measurements and use the largest)

On the table will be a growth chart for 'Boys 0-4 years'. The candidate will be given all the measurements (after advising which ones they would like) and asked to plot them and thus calculate the centiles. The measurement must be plotted using a pencil and as a single dot, not a cross.

After 6 minutes please stop the candidate and ask them the following questions:

What action might you take with this child and why?

Answer: They have dropped two centiles in weight and therefore need further assessment for potential failure to thrive.Give three causes of failure to thrive:

Any of:
1.   Poor nutritional intake/dietary (e.g. inappropriate feeding, poverty, maternal factors etc)

2. Inadequate nutrient absorption or increased losses (e.g. malabsorption, vomiting, infectious causes)
3. Increased nutrient requirements (e.g. chronic conditions-congenital heart disease, CF, hyperthyroidism etc)
4. Social or emotional abuse
5. Endocrine causes (e.g. hypothyroidism, hypoadrenalism, pituitary disorders)

Actor's Instructions:

You have brought your 13-month-old son to the hospital after being referred by your nurse practitioner who is concerned about his weight gain.

He was born at 41 weeks by emergency caesarean section for failure to progress but was born in good condition. He weighed 3.7kg at birth (25th-50th centiles) and his head circumference was 35.5cm (50th centile). He was a 'low risk' pregnancy and you were well throughout.

Apart from losing weight in the first 10 days he has been growing along the 50th centile and was last weighed aged 10 months. He was exclusively breast-fed until 6 months when you began introducing solids. He now eats three meals a day with some breast-feeds. He has had several admissions to hospital over the past 3 months with chest infections and wheeze and intermittently vomits. Otherwise he has no medical problems.

CLINICAL SKILLS – GROWTH CHARTS

Task:	Achieved	Not Achieved
Introduces self to patient/parent		
Checks correct patient name, date of birth and address		
Gains consent from parent for weight/length/head circumference measurements		
Advises child should be weighed whilst undressed and without a nappy		
Advises length should be measured without a nappy and using a measuring board/mat		
Advises head circumference to be measured 3 times and the largest reading taken		
Selects appropriate "Boys 0-4 years" growth chart		
Correctly fills in patient's details on growth chart		
Plots 'birth parameters' accurately for comparison		
Plots weight correctly		
Determines centile (9th)		
Plots length correctly		
Determines centile (25th)		
Plots head circumference correctly		
Determines centile (50th)		
Plots parameters using pencil and single dot		
Recognises fall in centiles represents faltering growth		
Suggests examining Red Book for previous growth parameters		
Offers three causes for faltering growth		
Explains everything clearly to parent and avoids medical jargon		
Examiner's Global Mark	/5	
Actor / Helper's Global Mark	/5	
Total Station Mark	/30	

Learning Points

There is no single threshold below which a child's height or weight is definitely 'abnormal', but children growing below the 0.4th centile should definitely be assessed in order to exclude any potential problems.

A child's growth may fluctuate above and below a centile but what is important is their general 'growth trend'. If a child's weight does fall by two or more centiles then a thorough assessment should be made.

Don't be caught out when plotting growth parameters for premature babies. Remember that plotting with gestational correction should be:
Until 1 year for infants born between 32-36 weeks,
Up to 2 years for infants born less than 32 weeks.

For further helpful tips and guidance on the UK-WHO growth charts please see the RCPCH website (Royal College of Paediatrics and Child Health 2016).

48. CLINICAL SKILLS - PRESCRIBING IMMUNISATIONS

Candidate's Instructions:

You are the FY1 on your GP rotation. An ex-32 week gestation baby, Bobby has been booked in to see you for their 12-week immunisations.

You are required to gain consent for and then prescribe, the appropriate vaccines as well as recording them in the 'Red Book'.

Examiner's Instructions:

The candidate is required to gain consent from the parent for their son's 12-week immunisations, which should include explaining common, rare and extremely rare side effects:

Common:
1. redness/swelling around injection site
2. Mild fever
3. Abnormal crying
4. Irritability

Rare:
1. high fever (>39°C)
2. Seizure activity

Extremely Rare:
 - Anaphylaxis

On the table is a blank drug chart and the candidate is required to prescribe the appropriate vaccines (5 in 1 and rotavirus), remembering to check for allergy status or any previous immunisation reactions. They should advise how the immunisations will be given (i.e. which site) and then record accurately in the 'Red Book'.

After 6 minutes please stop the candidate and ask them the following questions:

In what instances should immunisations be postponed?

> **Answer:**
>
> Febrile illness
>
> Signs of a worsening neurological problem/poorly controlled epilepsy.

When is the '5 in 1' vaccine absolutely contraindicated?
Answer:

Previous anaphylactic reaction to vaccine

Confirmed anaphylaxis to another component contained in the relevant vaccine

Why is it so important that premature babies in particular do not get behind on their immunisation programme?

Answer:
Being premature puts them at higher risk of catching infections.

Actor's Instructions:

You have brought your son, Bobby to the GP practice for his 12-week immunisations. He is currently well with no history of fever or recent illness.

Bobby was born at 32 weeks by emergency Caesarean section and was initially slow to feed but is now gaining weight well and your health visitor is happy.

You were discharged home 7 weeks ago and this is your second set of immunisations. The first set given at 8-weeks were quite traumatic as Bobby did not stop screaming. However, he did not have any severe reactions to the vaccines and you are happy for Bobby to have his 12-week set.

CLINICAL SKILLS - PRESCRIBING IMMUNISATIONS

Task:	Achieved	Not Achieved
Introduces self to parent		
Checks correct patient name, date of birth and address		
Gains consent for immunisations		
Ensures patient is well enough to receive immunisations today		
Ensures patient has had their previous immunisations (according to schedule)		
Correctly states would give '5 in 1' vaccine (Diptheria, Tetanus, Pertussis, Polio, Haemophilus influenza type B (Hib)		
Correctly states would give rotavirus vaccine		
Is aware that Men C vaccine is no longer given at 12 weeks *(ie. by stating or not prescribing)*		
Correctly fills out drug chart with patient details		
Correctly checks and records any allergy or previous drug reactions		
Correctly prescribes name of vaccine		
Correctly prescribes dose		
Correctly prescribes route (ensures '5 in1' given IM, and rotavirus given orally)		
Correctly states would inject the '5 in1' vaccine into the upper thigh		
Records immunisations have been given in the 'Red Book'		
Suggests when immunisations may be postponed		
Suggests contraindications to '5 in 1' vaccine		
Understands importance of immunisation to preterm infants		
Systematic approach to prescribing immunisations		
Explains everything clearly to parent and avoids medical jargon		
Examiner's Global Mark	/5	
Actor / Helper's Global Mark	/5	
Total Station Mark	/30	

Learning Points

Ensure you have a basic knowledge of the immunisation schedule for children. This can change from time to time so it is important to keep up to date (NHS Choices 2016).

Get into the habit in your history taking of asking about specific vaccines they should have had appropriate to their age, rather than asking whether they are 'up-to-date'. This is a safer way of ensuring no doses have been missed!

Some parents do not wish to vaccinate their children and our role as healthcare professionals is to try and educate them as to why it is so important. Try to engage these parents in meaningful conversations and always get advice from your seniors.

49. CLINICAL SKILLS - INTERPRET AN X-RAY OF A FRACTURE

Candidate's Instructions:

You are an FY1 doctor in the Emergency Department and have clerked a 9 year old boy who presented after falling onto his left hand whilst ice-skating.

He has returned from X-ray and your consultant would like you to interpret the radiograph and then present your findings to the medical student on your team in order to teach them about basic radiograph interpretation.

Please then discuss your differential causes followed by your management plan.

Examiner's/ Actor's Instructions:

The candidate will describe the fracture seen in the radiograph to the medical student and then discuss differential causes as well as their management plan.

The candidate should go through systematically how they would interpret and present a radiograph of a fracture. They must start with ensuring they have the correct patient film (patient name, hospital number and DOB) followed by stating the date, film type and adequacy. It is essential they advise that it is a 'left distal shaft radial fracture', with a transverse pattern and a degree of angulation.

After describing the fracture, the candidate should give their differential causes including: fall/trauma or non-accidental injury. They will then give a management plan including:

1.   Analgesia
2.   Senior Review
3.   Safeguarding check
4.   Surgical- likely need manipulation under anaesthetic
5.   Non-surgical- back slab + below elbow cast

Please stop them after 6 minutes and ask them to discuss their differential causes and management plan.

CLINICAL SKILLS STATION OSCE - Interpreting a Fracture

Task:	Achieved	Not Achieved
Introduces self to medical student		
Clarifies student's current level of knowledge of reporting fractures		
Checks radiograph has correct patient name		
Checks radiograph has correct date of birth		
Checks radiograph has correct hospital number		
Ensures correct date on the radiograph		
States that they are AP and lateral films of the radius and ulna, including the wrist and elbow joints.		
States the type of bone (i.e. radius)		
States the segment of bone (i.e. distal)		
States the pattern of the fracture (i.e. transverse)		
States that there is bone deformity (i.e. angulation)		
Suggests fracture may be caused by trauma eg., fall		
Suggests fracture may be a result of NAI		
Suggests giving analgesia		
Suggests senior ED / Orthopaedic review		
Suggests appropriate manipulation / casting of fracture		
States would ensure child had safeguarding check		
Summarises fracture and management plan concisely		
Systematic approach to radiograph interpretation		
Answers questions from medical student		
Examiner's Global Mark	/5	
Actor / Helper's Global Mark	/5	
Total Station Mark	/30	

Learning Points

Being able to have a systematic approach to interpreting fractures is crucial and will ensure you do not miss key features. Remember to report the date, name and type of film.

Developmental milestones are important when thinking of differential causes, as it is essential that the fracture be in keeping with the history for a child of that age. If you are not sure ALWAYS discuss with a senior for a child of any age and ensure a safeguarding check is completed.

All long bone fractures in a child <18 months should be highly suspicious for 'non accidental injury' and be discussed with an Emergency department or Paediatric consultant (Cardiff Child Protection Systematic Reviews 2016).

50. CLINICAL SKILLS - PRESCRIBING

Candidate's instructions

You are the paediatric FY1 in ED. Samira is a four day old baby who has been rushed in, critically ill with a fever and poor feeding. She is drowsy on examination. The working diagnosis is meningitis. You have been asked to prescribe intravenous antibiotics whilst the SHO gains intravenous access and the registrar manages her airway.

Samira is a term baby who was previously well, weighs 3.5 kg and has no allergies. Her full name is Samira Hussein, and her hospital number is H987654.

1. Prescribe appropriate iv antibiotics as per hospital protocol for Samira.

2. Prescribe iv maintenance fluids for Samira at 100 ml/kg/day.

3. In light of increasing concerns about raised intracranial pressure, change your iv fluid prescription to 2/3 maintenance fluids.

Examiner's instructions

You are the paediatric FY1 in ED. Samira is a four day old baby who has been rushed in, critically ill with a fever and poor feeding. She is drowsy on examination. The working diagnosis is meningitis. The candidate has been asked to prescribe intravenous antibiotics according to local hospital protocol.

The candidate is provided with a calculator, BNF for Children, a copy of the Trust antibiotic protocol and a blank drug chart.

Tasks given to candidate:

1.   Prescribe antibiotics.

1.   Prescribe intravenous maintenance fluids

1.   Change fluid prescription to 2/3 maintenance

DRUG CHARTS FOR PRESCRIBING

Name:		Hospital number:		DOB:		Weight:			
Allergies:				Signed:					
YEAR 20.... DATE AND MONTH →									
DOCTORS MUST ENTER administration times									
Date		Medication (print generic name)	TIMES						
Route	Dose	Frequency & (WRITE TIMES) →							
Indication / duration		Pharmacy							
Prescriber's signature	Print your name	Bleep							
Date		Medication (print generic name)	TIMES						
Route	Dose	Frequency & (WRITE TIMES) →							
Indication / duration		Pharmacy							
Prescriber's signature	Print your name	Bleep							
Date		Medication (print generic name)	TIMES						
Route	Dose	Frequency & (WRITE TIMES) →							
Indication / duration		Pharmacy							
Prescriber's signature	Print name	Bleep							

Name:	Hospital number:		DOB:	Weight:
Allergies:			Signed:	

Date	Fluid prescription	Route	Rate	Clinician	
	Infusion fluid & volume			Signature	Bleep
	Drug to be added			Print name	
	Infusion fluid & volume			Signature	Bleep
	Drug to be added			Print name	
	Infusion fluid & volume			Signature	Bleep
	Drug to be added			Print name	

TRUST PROTOCOL

Meningitis

Treatment if under one month of age:

Amoxicillin 100mg/kg IV twice a day (week one of life), three times a day (>1 week)
And cefotaxime 50mg/kg IV twice a day (week one of life), three times a day (>1 week)

Treatment if over one month of age and a previously healthy child:

Ceftriaxone 80 mg/kg (max 4g) IV daily

Treatment if over one month of age and with underlying diseases:

Meropenem (>1 month – 12 years and under 50 kg) 40mg/kg three times a day (>12 years or over 50kg) 2g three times a day.

CLINICAL SKILLS - PRESCRIBING

Task:	Achieved	Not Achieved
Legible block capitals and black pen used throughout		
Patient demographics (name / DOB / hospital number / weight / allergies) clearly entered		
Date / month written clearly on prescriptions		
All prescriptions signed with prescriber name		
Amoxicillin correctly selected		
Cefotaxime correctly selected		
Antibiotics indication specified (presumed meningitis)		
Antibiotics duration specified (e.g. 48 hours then review)		
Antibiotics administration times written in 24 hour clock in left hand grey column (e.g. 10:00 and 22:00)		
Antibiotics dose calculation entered (100 mg/kg and 50 mg/kg respectively)		
Amoxicillin dose 350 mg		
Amoxicillin frequency twice daily		
Cefotaxime dose 175 mg		
Cefotaxime frequency twice daily		
Safe fluid chosen (10% dextrose or 0.9% saline & 5% dextrose)		
Volume = bag volume (500ml)		
Nil added in 'drugs to be added' column		
Rate at 100 ml/kg/day = 15 ml/hr		
2/3 maintenance = 10 ml/hr		
New prescription written for new fluid rate (NOT adjustment of original prescription)		
Examiner's Global Mark	/5	
Total Station Mark	/25	

Learning points

Antibiotic doses, frequencies and antimicrobial agent often significantly vary across the paediatric population according to both the types of pathogen likely responsible and the differing pharmacokinetics applying to different age groups.

IV fluids used most commonly for maintenance fluid in paediatric populations are as follows:
    10% dextrose (neonatal population, at >24 hours of life will need bespoke sodium and potassium added to the bag according to blood electrolyte results)
    0.9% sodium chloride and 5% dextrose plus 10 mmol potassium chloride in each 500 ml bag (all other children apart from in very specialised situations)

IV fluid requirements for maintenance fluids are calculated by weight as follows
    First 10kg – 100 ml/kg
    Second 10 kg – 50 ml/kg
    Each subsequent kg – 20 ml/kg

Therefore a 25 kg child will need 1000 ml + 500 ml + 100 ml = 1600 ml per day. Divide this by 24 hours to calculate 66 ml/hour as the iv fluid rate. 2/3 maintenance fluids are often used in situations high risk for raised intracranial pressure or SIADH e.g. LRTI, asthma, meningitis.

References

British Thoracic Society, 2016. British Guideline on the Management of Asthma. *Thorax*.

Cardiff Child Protection Systematic Reviews, 2016. Fractures. Available at: http://www.core-info.cardiff.ac.uk/reviews/fractures.

EPICure, 2006. EPICure2. Available at: http://www.epicure.ac.uk.

HeadSmart, 2016. HeadSmart. Available at: www.headsmart.org.uk.

National Institute for Health and Care Excellence, 2016. Feverish illness in children overview. , (June).

National Perinatal Epidemiology Unit, 2010. UK TOBY Cooling Register Clinician's Handbook. , (May), p.24. Available at: https://www.npeu.ox.ac.uk/tobyregister/docs.

NHS Choices, 2016. When to have vaccinations. Available at: http://www.nhs.uk/conditions/vaccinations/Pages/vaccination-schedule-age-checklist.aspx.

Resuscitation Council UK, 2015. Paediatric advanced life support. Available at: https://www.resus.org.uk/resuscitation-guidelines/paediatric-advanced-life-support/.

Resuscitation Council UK, 2016. The ABCDE approach. Available at: https://www.resus.org.uk/resuscitation-guidelines/abcde-approach/.

Royal College of Paediatrics and Child Health, 2016. RCPCH UK-WHO Growth Charts, 0-18 years. Available at: http://www.rcpch.ac.uk/Research/UK-WHO-Growth-Charts.

Sarnat, H. & Sarnat, M., 1976. Neonatal encephalopathy following fetal distress. A clinical and electroencephalographic study. *Archives of Neurology*, 33(10), pp.696–705.

Printed in Great Britain
by Amazon